KILLING CANCER

The Jason Winters Story

by

Benjamin Roth Smythe

DISTRIBUTED
by
NUTRI BOOKS

VINTON PUBLISHING
1244 Wyoming Street
Boulder City, Nevada 89005

© BENJAMIN ROTH SMYTHE 1980

1st printing 1980
2nd printing 1980
3rd printing 1981
4th printing 1982
5th printing 1982
6th printing 1982
7th printing 1982
8th printing 1982
9th printing 1983
10th printing 1983

ISBN 0 7050 0096 6

1 2 3 4 5 6

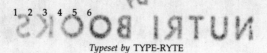

Typeset by TYPE-RYTE

THE JASON WINTERS' FAMILY

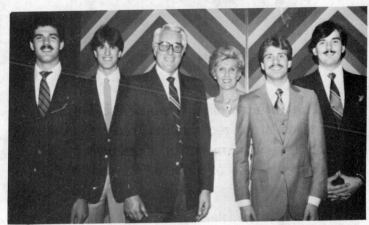

They all quit school and started work to help support the family—now in perfect health.

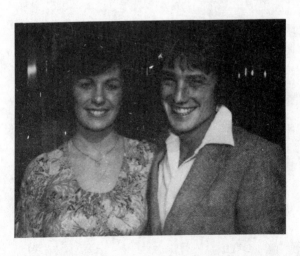

Daughter Cathy and Son-in-law Kerry

The author wishes to make it clear that he does not recommend total rejection of orthodox methods of cancer treatment – or a doctor's advice.

KILLING CANCER

Introduction

When I was first contacted by Jason Winters to write about his experiences I was very busy with other writings, and even though he was calling from the U.S.A. I tried to put him off. He was quite persistent however, and finally I told him to send me the manuscript for my perusal. Within a week a package arrived and it consisted of cassette tapes, entitled *"The Jason Winters Story."* I listened to them with complete dis-interest, then sat up and started to take notice. Something in this man's voice portrayed sincerity and great compassion.

His claims about cancer, herbs, laetrile, world travel and ultimate health, if true, were something the world should know about without delay.

First though, I had to check out his story, the hospital, doctors, x rays, cancer clinic, Dr. Malcolm Rea of Great Britian, and others. Then I started to check his source of information, starting with the Bible, the writing of Buddha, Krishna, Bihii Ulla, and Hippocretes. Everything I found verified Winters' story.

The checking took me six months, then I informed Winters that I would indeed write this little book for him. As always, I have written in the first person.

The book gives information about a trio of herbs that were mixed together into a tea. However, in 1981, Winters along with a few other well known Englishmen found that a capsul consisting of the original herbs and the spice plus additions was more convenient than the tea. The English have known for centuries that ingesting the whole herb is far more beneficial than making a tea and then throwing the leaves (herbs) away.

And so, dear reader, I give you The Jason Winters Story, part one. May it be an inspiration to all whom read it.

Benjamin Roth Smythe

Author.

WARNING: Please do not buy any Jason Winters Products from any source (including health food stores) until you contact Jason Winters. Crooks are already cashing in on your misfortune by selling useless products & using Jason Winters name & photo.

Contents

Preface

And God said, "Behold, I have given you every herb bearing seed which is upon the face of all the earth, and every tree in which is the fruit of a tree yielding seed: to you it shall be for meat." *Gen 1:29*

"And the fruit thereof shall be for meat, and the leaf thereof for medicine." *Ezekial 47:12*

"He causeth the grass to grow for cattle, and herbs for the use of man." *Psalm 104:14*

"For one believeth he may eat all things; another who is weak eateth herbs." *Romans 14:2*

"And the leaves of the trees were for the healing of nations." *Revelation 22:2*

But powerful man-made organizations today tell us:

What does God know? What does Buddha know? What does Hippocretes know? Eat aspirins, Bufferins, Valium, and after the side effects of these have caused worse problems, have chemotherapy. When your hair falls out, buy a wig. I will give you prescriptions to deaden the pain, allow you to go through life like a Zombie, and when you are too sick for us to help you anymore, then go home and prepare to die.

But, if you should obtain help from a herbalist, nutritionist, or any other than a doctor of medicine, then we will persecute him, if he makes you well, and prosecute him, if you should die like the doctor said you would.

If you live, then we will laugh at you and harass you, and tell you that you were never ill in the first place.

I believe that if Jesus were to suddenly appear in America today to heal people, He would be arrested for practicing medicine without a license. Telling people that they can be healed by proper eating, thinking and living would result in an immediate jail sentence.

They would not make Him walk the streets this time carrying a cross, but would rather crucify Him in all the establishment newspapers and other media. They would harass and ridicule Him, and they would drive Him out of the country.

For Jesus to help us in America today, He would have to live in the safety of Mexico, where all who wish to help people the natural way are forced to go.

Jason Winters

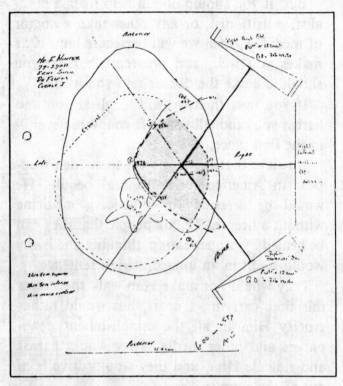

This is a medical drawing of Jason Winters' head based on actual X-ray photos. The view is from the top of the skull looking down. The shaded area marks the tumor.

1. Terminal Cancer

I walked into the Cobalt Radiation Department for the first time and was filled with despair. This department took care of patients suffering from head and neck cancer. There were about 20 patients in the waiting room, and I took my place among them. My heart was thumping, and with good reason, for the faces all around me showed fear and depression. I could smell death in the air. Most of the people had hardly any hair left, due to the chemotherapy treatment. Ash-trays were scattered around the room and nearly everyone was smoking heavily. When I mentioned that smoking is bad for health, one patient said, 'Well, it's too late for us now anyway, isn't it?'

One by one patients had their names

called and would disappear behind a large lead door. When they came out they looked worse than before – and left hurriedly. I was worried as I had no idea what was behind that door. Would I too, soon have no hair and that look of terror in my eyes? I heard the nurse call my name, and as if in a daze found myself following her into the treatment room.

I had first noticed the swelling on the side of my neck when taking a steam bath at the Y.M.C.A. Although 46 years old I was in top physical condition – running and swimming each day. Life was a ball for me, for I had a great wife, five nice kids and a good income. I smoked 30 cigarettes a day, and did some real hard drinking at least once a week. Rye whiskey was my favourite.

The lump seemed to ache deep inside my throat but I was not worried. I bought some lozenges and tried to forget about it. As the days went by the lump got bigger and bigger, but I avoided my doctor like the plague. I was unconsciously scared of what the lump might be. After a few more weeks even my friends noticed the swelling and remarked on it. I realised that I could not avoid the issue indefinitely, so I made an appointment with our family doctor.

He at once sent me to a surgeon. It resulted in dozens of x-rays, examinations at the Nuclear Medicine Center, scans, pills – and fear. At last it was decided that I must go into hospital to have a small biopsy operation. The surgeon said it would take only half an hour and result in a scar a couple of inches long.

Soon after I checked into the hospital a dear old lady came around with lots of strong black coffee, white sugar and cream buns. She was trying hard to serve humanity, and no one ever told her she was serving what I later found out to be the very worst things a cancer patient, or anyone else for that matter, can eat and drink.

When I awoke from the operation I found that it had taken six and a half hours, and left a scar nine inches long. I saw immediately that my wife had been crying. I guess that was when I first knew for sure my condition was serious. The doctor walked in and said, 'Terminal cancer. Infiltrating squamous cell carcinoma'. The tumor was wrapped around my carotid artery and, to make matters even worse, was attached to the wall of my jugular vein.

After telling me three times that my condition was terminal, the doctor left me to my misery. My wife Jan went home to break the news to our five children. Thoughts of death crowded in on me from all sides. Reading, television, radio were all drowned out by the thoughts that soon I would be gone.

The next morning, when my doctor made his rounds, he did not find me in bed. Another patient and I were having a hilarious pillow fight from our wheel-chairs. The doctor was furious. 'Don't you know you have terminal cancer? Don't you realise you should be in bed?' Because I was sure that all doctors are gods, I obeyed him quickly. But it was not long before I was out of bed again – this time to trudge around the hospital.

I walked around the whole place five times for exercise, and when I returned it was the head nurse's turn to be furious. She said the doctor had been complaining to her about me, and once again assured me that I had terminal cancer, and must at least stay in my room.

It seemed to me that everyone was worried in case I forgot to die. The doctor even went so far as to lecture my wife on my behaviour. 'Doesn't he know he's got terminal cancer? Doesn't he believe me?' Many tests followed and finally it was agreed what my treatment should be. I would have five weeks of cobalt radiation on my neck and head, and then if the swelling were down, I could have radical neck surgery. That meant the removal of my tongue, jaw bone, neck muscles and also the inside of my throat. To begin with I would receive three cobalt treatments each day for five weeks.

I felt better as soon as I left the hospital and walked down the street. I felt free, even though I got a lot of stares from people gaping at the bandages around my face and neck. At least they couldn't see the tumor.

My first appointment with the cancer clinic did not bother me too much. I had to be fitted for a plastic mask. This went right over my head like the Count of Monte Cristo mask. There were three holes in one side for it to be attached to the cobalt machine, so that I could not move my head while being bombarded with radiation. I had to go back in one week for another fitting, and this really depressed me. I got so bad that I would not let my wife tell anyone that I had cancer. I could not stand the look of fear in their faces and the way even old friends changed towards me. I would not even let my children say the word cancer. That shows how bad I had become.

The nurse in the cobalt room called my name – and it had started.

For five weeks I was to see my fellow patients gradually get weaker and weaker – then I would see them no more. One friend was a big strong man and had a tumor on the side of his head. After many cobalt treatments his right eye started running, so they *sewed it closed*. I will always remember the terror in his one good eye, as he looked at me in desperation. I said, 'Don't worry, we will both get better', not believing it myself of course. My friend beamed and he shouted to all the other patients, 'Did you hear that? Jason says we are both going to get better.' It was many months later that I understood what he meant and why he was so happy. Since he had discovered he had cancer, he had been told repeatedly, 'Terminal, terminal'. I was the first one in the whole wide world to tell him he would get better, or to offer even any hope at all. He died two days later. I started taking 10 valium tablets each day, so that I would not break down and cry, as well as six pain pills and six sleeping pills.

The cobalt treatment took away my taste, made it impossible for me to make saliva, burned the right side of my face and made my hair on that side fall out. Life was hell.

I went from 263 lbs down to 170 lbs. My knees were shaky and I could not stay awake for longer than four hours at a time. It was then that I discovered the value of pure honey and vitamin E. As I would sit on the couch in shock, after the cobalt treatment, I would eat spoonfuls of honey. I could not taste it but I knew it was good for me. I stopped losing weight. I smeared the vitamin E on my burned face, and soon there was a great improvement. Doctors at the cancer clinic remarked how well I was taking the treatment. I told them what I was doing and they said that this was fine, but I was not to mention it to the others.

That remark puzzled me no end. I thought about it constantly. I *did* tell the others about it and they all started the same treatment with good results. But the doctors did not want me to tell anyone about it. The only answer I could figure out to this scared the heck out of me, but it probably saved my life. I started to realize that doctors are not gods after all. Maybe they can make mistakes too. If that was right then maybe they had made a mistake about me. They all kept telling me to get my affairs in order, and prepare to die, but perhaps I didn't have to die.

The next day the surgeon called me into his office. He had decided to operate on me as soon as possible. Radical neck surgery. Removal of tongue, jaw bone and neck muscles. He went into great detail about the operation. When I asked him if I would live any longer from having the surgery, he said probably not. I looked him straight in the eye and said, '*No*'. The doctor said, 'What do you mean, No?' I said, 'No operation'. Then I stood up and walked out of his office. My heart was singing. I was going to keep my tongue and die in one piece.

Many times the doctor called my wife to tell her to get me into hospital. Everyone was trying to get me there, even though everyone knew that I-would die anyway. I couldn't understand it. I wondered who these people thought they were, asking me to have this terrible operation.

Then I heard about laetrile.

2. Laetrile

I heard that laetrile was made from apricot kernels and contained a little cyanide, necessary in our body in small amounts. I went at once to the health food store and bought six bottles of apricot kernels. I would eat about 50 a day. Soon the aching stopped and it looked as though the tumor was actually shrinking. I was elated and overjoyed. I did not worry about being cured. Just as long as I could keep it under control would be good enough for me.

When I ran out of the kernels I returned to the health food store for more. I was told that the government authorities had removed them from the shelves. I was horrified. How could anyone do this? The man in the health food store offered a possible explanation. Laetrile could control cancer without all the operations and radiation that I had been through. What would happen to those people who work in cancer clinics by the thousands? They would be unemployed of course. Drug companies would lose millions, as would doctors, surgeons, anaesthetists and nurses. 30 major countries of the world use laetrile in the treatment of cancer, but in North America it was banned.

Now I had not yet got over the fact that doctors could make mistakes, so it took a lot of thought and investigation before I could realize the monstrous evil behind banning apricot kernels and laetrile. Dying people are sent home with the words, 'We can't do anything for you', without the right even to try the biggest natural cancer fighter of all time.

I heard that the Contreras Clinic in Tijuana, Mexico, gave laetrile to patients, and my heart leapt. My wife and family made arrangements to accompany me, and off we went to Mexico.

We arrived at Centro Medico Del Mar in Tijuana early in the morning, and were soon surrounded by hundreds of Americans and Canadians all in the same position as myself. However there was a difference from the other cancer clinics, for here I could see hope and enthusiasm shining on everyone's faces. After a complete examination by a doctor I was scheduled for laetrile injections each day and also put on a diet. I felt better already. For the first time in my life I started eating sensibly. Part of the cure must be correct diet. Slowly I started building up my body. I thought of the old lady at the hospital with her coffee, white sugar and cream buns – all definite taboos at the clinic. Almost everyone here had a miraculous story to tell. I was slowly emerging from that long black tunnel of death, and I was ecstatic.

All of the patients here were terminal patients from the U.S. and Canada that had exhausted every avenue of orthodox treatment and now were trying this as a last resort. But miracles were happening here, and I thanked God that I had heard about it.

Each morning I would join in the line with hundreds of patients and when my turn came I would go into a cubicle and receive an enzyme enema. Right after this would come the laetrile injection. I can honestly say that there were no adverse effects experienced either by myself or any of the others. In ten days the tumor had shrunk to half the size and the doctor stated that I could return home, but must take some laetrile tablets with me. I should take these three times each day. He said that my cancer was under control. I emerged from the clinic a happy man, hardly able to believe my good fortune.

When I arrived home I found that the cancer clinic had called many times. They wanted me to go up in front of a panel of doctors to be examined. They were all sure that I would have to have the operation. They knew nothing of my trip to Mexico.

I arrived early for the examination, anxious to see the expression on their faces when they discovered the tumor almost gone. One by one they examined me. But not one of them said a word to me. There were no smiles, no congratulations, no happiness at all. When I finally told them I had been taking laetrile, the doctor who had wanted to remove my tongue and so on said that I could not have had cancer in the first place. Another said he must perform the operation anyway. I was horrified at the way these people acted, and left as soon as possible.

I thought the doctors would be overjoyed that my tumor had gone, would demand to know how I had done it, then hold press conferences around the world, stating just what happened. I thought of the thousands who were waiting for cobalt treatment, or were swallowing chemotherapy poison, so bad for the system it makes the patients' hair fall out, makes them vomit continually and fills the body full of toxins. I thought of the thousands who were waiting to enter the operating rooms of hospitals around the country, waiting to have colostomies and tumors removed. Terrible operations that removed the effects but not the cause. I

thought of all the thousands who that very
week would be told they had cancer, and of
how they would start dying immediately,
because to them just the word cancer meant
certain death. I felt like running through
every cancer clinic in North America shout-
ing that there is a control for cancer. Don't
let that little old lady fill your ailing bodies
with poisonous coffee and white sugar. Start
eating God's health foods right now.

3. Nutrition

Now I know for sure that some readers are just as naive as I was about cancer, the medical profession, laetrile and all alternative therapies. I know that some people are so stubborn that they would die rather than admit they are wrong, and often do. If it's only your own life at stake, do as you wish, but if you are concerned with someone else's life, such as a loved one, a friend or relative, then remember, you are not God, and they deserve the benefit of the doubt. The whole reason for this book is to make you have a doubt, then maybe you will search for the truth.

'Things that are sweet in the mouth are bitter in the stomach.' We know that too much sugar and sweet things are bad for us. And things that are bitter in the mouth may be sweet in the stomach. Bitter almonds and apricot kernels are very bitter, and this is what laetrile is made from. God wants us to be healthy, so he gave us everything we need to live long healthy lives. In this age of people proudly stating 'My son the doctor' I fear that we have made doctors our gods. It is interesting to note that in Oden's book, *Thank God I have Cancer*, it is shown that doctors and their families are among the unhealthiest in the nation. I quote:

10% already have cancer.
12% already have anaemia.
21% have allergies.
24% have had major surgery.
30% are overweight.

These are the people that we run to with our sick bodies. These are the people we run to, instead of God. By the thousands we rush to psychiatrists, asking them to straighten out our minds. In reality, psychiatrists have the highest suicide rate of any group in the world. These are facts. Once in a while it is possible to find a doctor who works with nature and with God. This person will rely mainly on natural foods, vitamins and minerals to help your body regain health. When he performs surgery it is necessary. Find a doctor who believes God is greater than the medical associations, and you have found a jewel.

He will suggest you eat properly, he may well recommend B17 (laetrile) because he will be unbiased and really care about you. He makes no money from laetrile, and there is not a drug salesman giving him free samples. This man cares so much because God is his boss – not a medical association. I feel that medical associations are like unions; designed to keep their members busy and financially secure. Can you name a nation other than America where a doctor expects to make hundreds of thousands of dollars each year? Can you name another country where doctors will not make house calls? Where they expect to retire at such an early age? Where they will charge you for not showing up for an appointment, but can keep you waiting for hours? Do they make money from sickness or health? Supposing that eating properly, along with God's natural immunity that He has given us all, kept everyone healthy, what would happen to the biggest business in America today?

It is interesting to note that in some provinces of China a doctor is paid, by the government, a flat fee each month. When anyone gets sick, the doctor is fined a small amount. You see, he failed to keep his people healthy. He makes money out of health, whereas our doctors only can survive if we keep getting ill.

Find a God-loving, nutritionally conscious doctor and you may avoid the treadmill of death. That is what I call orthodox cancer treatment. First the radiation which burns and sears, then the operation which removes the effect and not the cause, which also leaves you weak and in shock, and finally, if you have survived this, you are given chemotherapy. You are ill because your body is full of poisons, but now they are pouring more down your throat. Poison so drastic that sometimes they have to stop the treatment for a while so you can get stronger. Imagine a medicine so toxic that they have to take you off of it so that you will get stronger by yourself. You have suffered all of this and yet God's system is still working within you. But oh, how it needs help. Nutrition. A change of mind about cancer. Yes, the treadmill of death. If you are an American, from the time you are told you have cancer until you die, you will have spent an average of seventeen thousand five hundred dollars. A doctor told me that once he or his associates discover cancer in a patient, they mentally write him off. He is as good as dead. I think doctors convey this attitude of helplessness to the patient.

Now I am a firm believer in mind over matter. So that if you have made a god of your doctor, then you will certainly do what he tells you, even to the extent of dying as expected. After all, faith can move mountains. Then why shouldn't you die when

your medical god tells you that you should?
It is hard to change from a negative to a
positive attitude, especially when you have
been bombarded with radiation, cut up with
surgery and then poisoned with chemotherapy. But talk to the thousands of people
at the laetrile clinics in Mexico and Germany. They all go to these clinics after the
medical profession has given up on them.
My telling you what is taking place there
every day is not enough. You must take full
responsibility for your own life. You must
find out this exciting truth for yourself.

Some people of course are so stubborn
that they cannot be helped. Although it is
heart-breaking there is nothing you can do.
The following story is a typical example.

Two young boys, one ten years old and
one seven had identical tumors in the left
leg. The seven year old's parents were well
aware of nutritional cures. When told that
major surgery was necessary they refused,
and the boy was put on a nutritional diet
and laetrile. Six weeks later the tumor was
gone and he has complete remission. His

smiling happy face is a glorious sight to behold.

However, the ten year old's parents believed that if there was a cure for cancer then the doctors would know about it. When they asked their doctor about laetrile he called it a useless toxic hoax, used by charlatans and quacks.

As of this writing the little boy is waiting for his third operation. He has already lost his left leg. His hair has fallen out. My heart goes out to him and to the thousands of others on this medically approved treadmill of death.

Can you imagine what would happen if suddenly the truth were to come out? As Red Buttons, the comedian said, to reporters of the *National Enquirer*, 'People who suppress laetrile, and stop other people from using it are nothing more than murderers.' Buttons' wife gained remission of cancer through laetrile.

Fred McMurray of T.V. fame gained remission of cancer through laetrile. A won-

derful man who said No to orthodox methods
and took the natural way back to health.

People involved in laetrile have been
persecuted. Many have been taken to court,
won the case, only to be taken to court again
and again. This is harassment. Even though
a person wins every case, he can go broke
just defending himself. So the million dollar
drug cartels win after all. One top doctor
told me that as long as more people benefit
from cancer than suffer from it, we will be
happy to go along just like this. Hundreds
of millions are spent on cancer research
each year, providing many top paying jobs.
A startling fact to remember in all of this is
that statistics indicate that one person in
four will have cancer next year. No wonder,
the way we are eating and drinking junk.
No wonder our bodies are fighting a losing
battle.

In spite of all the persecutions and har-
assments, those pushing for the right of
patients to use laetrile are winning. We can
now obtain laetrile (B17 or amygdalin) in
most states and provinces, although it's not

easy, and it is expensive. It is estimated that three thousand people in Canada alone order laetrile every month. They have to order it from Germany or Mexico because the home made stuff is not always pure. The average person spends about one hundred dollars each month on laetrile, which means that over three hundred thousand dollars each month are leaving a country with a population of just twenty million.

To get an idea of how much Americans are spending on laetrile each month, just multiply that figure by ten. Laetrile is a God-given vitamin that attacks cancer cells and is completely non-toxic if obtained in its pure form.

Should the powers that be in North America make it difficult for the millions of people destined to get cancer in the next few years to obtain laetrile? The largest manufacturer of laetrile in Europe ships out over five hundred thousand orders each month to doctors, hospitals, clinics and patients all over the world. Also, laetrile in the form of bitter almonds and apricot kernels has been in use to fight tumors for 4000 years. Recently, while browsing through a book store in London, I was surprised to come across a book, first published in 1810 and written by Jacob Antworth. On page 81 he states that in order to eliminate growths, the kernels from apricots should be crushed and mixed with your morning oats! You will be glad to know that God did not put all His eggs in one basket, so to speak. The following foods all contain laetrile: alfalfa, buckwheat, cassava, flaxseed, broad beans, lima beans, garlic, soya beans, berries, blackstrap molasses, macademia nuts, sprouts, rye, rice, bran, peas, oats, millet and the seeds of apple, plum, cherry and of course apricot. So start helping yourselves to God's way of killing cancer. Pancreatic enzymes are also very important to the cancer patient. Two tablets taken prior to laetrile allow the latter to work more effectively. It seems that the enzymes rush to the cancerous area where they start eating away at the protein shell that usually surrounds and protects a tumor. This allows the laetrile to penetrate the tumor and release its cyanide onto the cancer cells to kill them.

When you remember that all natural means were given us by God, it means that the authorities have rejected God's methods. I think that everyone knows that if you are for God, then you are spiritual, and if you are against God then you are evil.

Americans told by their doctors to prepare to die are filling clinics in Mexico and Germany, and many are going home in a few weeks with their cancer in complete remission. These clinics are not run by quacks either. Most of the world's foremost cancer scientists believe that laetrile is a wonderful anti-cancer agent. Among them are Dr. N. R. Boujiane of Montreal, Dr. John Morrone, New Jersey, Dr. Hans Nieper, Germany, Dr. Contreras of Mexico and Dr. Navarro of Manilla. Of course the findings of such men are discounted in America. They dare to take a different stand, and so are often ridiculed. Jesus was persecuted for being different, and Giordano Bruno was burned at the stake for teaching that the world is round. Laetrile works in many, many cases and is certainly worth a try. It takes away the pain and makes one far more comfortable.

I have spoken to hundreds of people who should have died twenty years ago, according to their doctors, but they discovered laetrile and have taken it daily ever since and are as healthy as can be. I have gone into the laetrile story at great lengths because I am about to shock you, and before I do I want you to know that laetrile works for thousands of people.

My tumor started coming back. I was taking the enzymes and the three thousand milligrams of laetrile every day, but the swelling started coming back. In shock, I increased the dosage but it did no good whatsoever.

After three weeks the tumor was as big as it was before, so I called the laetrile clinic. I was told that this sometimes but rarely happens, and there was not much that I could do. I was on a strict diet of fruit and vegetables with large doses of vitamins, but it was getting worse.

Now I really did live with death 24 hours each day. It was as though I had been given life, only to have it snatched away. This time I really did prepare to die. I purchased all kinds of religious books and while my family went to work to keep groceries on the table I read them all. In my misery I was struck by how many times herbs are mentioned in the Bible, even on the first page. Herbs as medicines show up in so many different religions that it seemed to be too much of a coincidence. Hippocrates, father of medicine, stated that herbs shall be for medicine. So did Buddha and Krishna. Then I found that the North American Indians believed in herbs and used them as medicine; also the gypsies of Europe, and the Hunzas, and the aborigines. All spiritual writings somewhere or other mention herbs for healing.

In desperation my mind cast about to decide what I should do. It would be so easy to do nothing, and to waste away. I was full of dread and fatigue. But I could not die yet. Besides, I was too scared to die. I must find the herbs that God put here for this purpose. And so started a search around the world.

4. Healing Herbs

Once I started learning about herbs as
medicine I did become a little excited, but
not much, especially after my let down with
laetrile. The most powerful ancient herb for
tumors seemed to come from Asia. I went to
every herbalist in my area, then telephoned
others across the country. They had never
heard of it except in old books from Asia.
The more difficult this herb became for me
to find the more determined I was that I had
to have it.

When I learned that it was available in
Singapore, I started thinking about travelling there. The only problem was money.
We had six thousand dollars to our name,
did not own a house or anything else worth
while that I could get a loan on. Also we had
five kids to support. But still, we all felt that

this was a matter of life and death. My eldest child went to stay with friends, and my sixteen and fifteen year old sons quit school (we hoped, temporarily) and got jobs. I had many credit cards left over from my more affluent days and I figured I would use these to pay travel expenses. If I survived then I would pay them back, and if not, my wife would have to declare bankruptcy. So it came about that with our two youngest children, my wife and I boarded a plane – destination Singapore. The fact that my two children had to support me, one under each arm, caused the Singapore immigration some concern. For a moment it was touch and go on whether they would let me into the country. We explained that I was merely airsick, which I am sure they did not believe, as the tumor was obvious to all. They decided in our favour and we soon found ourselves at the hotel. My wife lost no time in looking for the herb, which was not available in the stores in Singapore. At last she came upon an old lady living a distance from town, who cultivated the herb. Evidently she dug up the roots and boiled 50 lbs in a large container. After boiling vigorously for 26 hours, she was left with a liquid concentrate which she sold for a very high price. Usually sold in half ounce bottles, she was surprised when we asked for one pint. I was told it would definitely get rid of my cancer. I can remember that I held that bottle with great reverence; after all, this is the very thing that the great Buddha suggested for tumors. I could hardly wait to get back to the hotel to start drinking it. The directions were to take one eighth of a teaspoonful in a large glass of water, once each day, until well.

For ten days I took the medicine, and when nothing happened I doubled the dose. The tumor, although not getting any bigger stayed the same size exactly. A hurried visit to the old lady brought merely a shrug. She had no idea why it had not worked. She said, 'Well at least it's stopped growing' and that was it. My wife insisted that we buy another pint from her, even though we still had a lot left over. Jan was so impressed by the old lady's knowledge that she figured even if it did not cure cancer, it would prevent her getting it. Both her parents had died of the disease.

We left Singapore feeling very low indeed. I felt the herb did not work, and maybe that was why it didn't. We left for our next destination which was Tucson, Arizona.

Years before I had been a stunt man and a bit actor in Hollywood. We had made a few films with Audie Murphy in a place called Old Tucson, just a few miles from Tucson. Old Tucson was built in the old western style for Hollywood. Many western movies were made there, including 'Apache Agent', in which I played. I had learned at that time about a tea which most Indians, especially Mexican Indians, drank for health, and that's what prompted our visit. In Arizona we soon located the herb, known as chaparral, or the creosote bush (divaricata). Once again we heard that this remedy had been passed down through the ages and would prevent or get rid of cancer.

We stayed at the Santa Rita Hotel in

Tucson then moved to a small motel with a kitchen. The chaparral tea which I had to make five times each day was putrid, and smelled as bad as it tasted. It was enough to make a healthy man sick, but I persisted. It seemed to do nothing at all, except make me sick, but looking back now I feel that although I was not getting better, I was not getting worse. But at the time, so obsessed with death and dying, I was too depressed to notice.

In Tucson, a nutritionist who learned of my condition, told us that in Europe there were many old remedies for different ills, even cancer. He said that because there is socialised medicine there (free doctors and hospitals), doctors don't expect to become rich over-night. Because of this they are more open to alternative inexpensive therapies. He said that if ever he became ill he would return to England for that reason alone. And so, as a last resort, we decided to visit England.

With five pounds of chaparral and a pint and a half of the Singapore potion we boarded the plane for London. We had already spent most of our cash and were now on credit cards. That was the only time in my life that I have ever appreciated credit.

Now I have dozens of relatives in England, but I would not let my wife contact any of them. I did not want them to see me like this, and I wanted no tears. This is the part of the trip that I enjoyed, because this was the country I was born in, and it did me good to see the beautiful countryside once more. In my heart I knew that the visit was not really necessary, but just returning home meant defeat, and going to England postponed the inevitable for a while.

Brome and Schimmer in the south of England are one of the biggest and most knowledgeable herbal companies in the world. They introduced me to red clover (Trifolium pratense), the gypsy health drink that is supposed to be good for many things. Evidently there is a big difference between red and white clover blossoms, with the white being inferior. White clover is sold all over North America as being the best.

Chopped up clover blossoms make a very nice tea, which I started drinking, also at the rate of five glasses each day. This meant that I was busy making tea all day, first with the Asian herb, then chaparral, then red clover.

On the fourth day I became very ill indeed. My legs were shaking and I felt terribly sick. I had to stay in bed. I stopped taking all the herbs and readied myself for death. Two days later I felt a little better and my wife Jan wanted to return home to Canada. This whole adventure had been very rough on her; she looked worn out, and wanted to return to whatever little security she had left. When we arrived our credit cards were promptly confiscated and we found we owed many thousands of dollars. Bill collectors were calling on the telephone and knocking on the door constantly; we were all very worried. My youngest son, Robin, was sent home from school because he broke down and started crying. When asked why, he said, 'My dad is dying of cancer'.

Healing Herbs

As a last resort, I started back on the herbal teas again. One morning, I can remember it well, I was at my lowest ebb. I thought to heck with it, I'll mix all the herbs together.

5. The Mixture

I was sick and tired of washing the tea pot all the time prior to making another type of herbal tea. It was five minutes to ten on a Wednesday morning. I made the tea combination and a miracle happened.

I could feel it with that first swallow. It seemed to ring a distant bell, a long past memory. It screamed at me that this was what I needed. Strength seemed to pour through my body. That day I made a gallon of the tea and drank it all. When my family walked through the door they could see the difference in my face. I was enthusiastic, excited and overjoyed. Tears filled all of our eyes. We did not understand what had happened but we all knew that something wonderful had taken place. Day after day I drank one gallon regularly. Strength and vitality returned, but mostly it was my frame of mind. I was going to live, I knew it. All depression left me, all morbid thoughts. The more excited I became the smaller the tumor got; the smaller the tumor became, the more I got excited. Within three weeks the tumor had gone completely. Everyone called it a miracle, because in nine weeks I returned to work. I was not as healthy as before, I was healthier, and God, how I enjoyed every minute of life.

My case became well known throughout the whole area and people with terminal cancer started lining up outside the door, just to talk to me. They all wanted the tea. Then my local priest called me into his office and said, 'Look Jason, I know and so do you that you have found something for cancer, and for other illnesses too. Why my haemorrhoids that I have suffered with for twenty years disappeared in two weeks of drinking your tea. Many other things are happening to people drinking it too. Good things. You have something here, and if you do nothing about it you can be guilty of the sin of omission. But, if you do decide to do something about it you can expect to be persecuted severely. The officials in North America won't let you ruin a multi-million dollar a year business without a fight, and they have the money, the power to ridicule you, and to threaten you.'

After much thought I decided to tell my story to the world. A small newspaper took up the story first, which resulted in over three hundred telephone calls and a thousand letters, plus a big line up outside the door, from eight a.m. until past midnight. My boss fired me because I was supposed to sell refrigerators, but cancer patients filled the store and we could not move. Everyone wanted the tea. Separately the herbs would not work for me; together they were a miracle. I started importing the ingredients and mixing them in four ounce bags, which I would give to anyone who wanted some. They in exchange would give a donation so that I could get more herbs.

The radio station told my story, which increased the customers tenfold. Never in the history of the radio station had they received so many calls as they did about that particular program.

One man with a brain tumor received such help that the doctors pronounced him well. Without my permission he had advertising made up about my tea. He wanted the world to know about it – he wanted to help everyone. He got me into trouble and my first persecutions began.

People started flying in to see me from Australia, Germany, and many other places in the world, and I was flooded under. The police became regular visitors to my place, making sure that I did not tell anyone that the herbs were any good for anything. But I didn't need to say anything. The world was so desperate for something natural that would work that I was constantly running out of herbs.

I started receiving many offers from people and companies, one even from a priest. I had never met this man before, but he came up to me and said, 'Take me in as your partner and we will make a million.

We can charge fifty dollars a four ounce bag, and I can get the hell out of this church.' All this, in front of a witness! I found it hard to believe, and told him a definite No.

Now the priest had in his congregation a particularly violent man who needed help desperately. The priest, mad at me for not accepting his offer, set this man on me. He actually attacked me once in the church. The priest would incite the man, whom I will call Mr. H. Strangely enough, one of the first letters reporting a cure was from Mr. H.'s wife. So furious were the priest and Mr. H. that they still to this day type letters to magazines and newspapers, and sometimes even to dying people, saying, 'Mr. Winters never had cancer, and if you want more information call Reverend . . .', and of course the letters are unsigned. So persecution and hatred come from various places. When a national magazine ran a 28 page story on my experiences and the tea, I thought it would be easy, but they took three months to put it together, and interviewed hundreds of people involved.

The Mixture

As far as the editors are concerned the tea works, and now they are steady drinkers of it themselves. At the time the article was being prepared, the Canadian version of the F.D.A. showed up and went through our files, taking the names of all our customers and confiscating all the tea we had. By this time I had three thousand people relying on me for the tea. They took up a collection and I left for Nassau in the Bahamas where I set up a company.

When the article came out in the magazine, we started receiving over 2000 orders each day, and that has continued with absolutely no advertising whatsoever. We had to hire all the unemployed people we could get to help us, and still the business grew. Over one thousand letters each month pour in telling of the relief and cures obtained from all kinds of ills. Hollywood stars, politicians, all types of medical men, attorneys, truck drivers, etc., order regularly.

Greed caused people to do some pretty terrible things. The priest previously mentioned, for instance. Knowing that I had left the country, he gathered a group of people around him and they are now selling a herbal mix, using my name, knowing that it is nowhere near the same tea. A health food distributor in Canada also could see the money in this, and is putting out a phony tea under my name. These people are of course trading lives for dollars, and I mention this so that the reader knows enough to be careful.

I have recently turned over the formula and all rights to the largest manufacturer of herbal preparations in England. The hatred, bitterness, greed and harassment proved too much for me to handle. Besides this, my values have changed. Money is not as important to me as being alive. I feel wonderful about life, and about God, who cured me. Greed and bitterness cause stress, and I think that stress causes cancer, so I will leave all those feelings behind.

6. Why the Tribalene Works

God placed a certain herb in each continent to cure illness by simply purifying the blood. Life is in the blood, and if anything purifies the blood then a person's God-given natural immunity will have a chance to take over and fight all disease.

It is as simple as that.

The herb God put in Asia will not grow elsewhere, and the same goes for chaparral of North America and red clover of Europe. If you try to grow these herbs elsewhere they do not thrive because of soil deficiencies.

Jesus spoke of one herb for purifying the blood, Buddha of another herb in Asia, and the North American spirit fathers of yet another. Now in those days, before coffee, white sugar, processed foods and fast food outlets, any one of these herbs would have done the trick on its own. However, we alive today have such toxic bodies that we don't know what good health really is; after all we have nothing to judge it by. Fed on canned milk from birth, then doctored up cow's milk, canned baby food, graduating to hamburgers, french fries, coffee and white poisonous sugar. That is why just one of these herbs would not work on me. I was so full of toxins, as you are, that it took the combined effort of three most powerful herbs to bring me back to health.

I did not know it at the time but while I was drinking the tea at first I became sick to my stomach. I should have noticed this as a good sign. All that was happening was that the herbs were clearing my body of poison, and it was taking place so fast that it was overpowering my liver. A good sign. What a patient should do in that case is take it easy for three days, then start on the herbs again. Eventually the body will be pure and you will not feel sick any more.

On a recent trip to England I was met

with open arms by the medical profession. They were anxious to try my tea. One radionics practitioner tested the tea with his machine and found that it raised his energy level from 47 to 88. This may not mean much to the average reader, but to anyone in the know about radionics it is quite astounding. We immediately got calls from reporters wanting interviews and these people were not the slightest bit hesitant about printing the facts about the tea. What a difference from America where the newspapers keep well away from anything like this, unless they are accusing you of something. Even the British royal family have their own herbalist, a Mrs. Blackie, who has treated the Queen and her family for years.

The highlight of my trip to England was meeting two wonderful men, Dr. Ian Pearce and Malcolm Rae. In Dr. Pearce we found a medical doctor with an open mind. I shall always remember sitting in his cottage in Norfolk listening to him talk about herbs. Mr. Rae on the other hand was one of the world's leading radionics practitioners. Sadly he died at the end of 1979. He placed the tea on a machine and startled us by saying that the tea worked not only on the physical level, but also on the mental and spiritual planes. Why this startled me is that the old lady in Singapore had said, 'This herb will bring the spiritual and mental bodies back into line with the physical body.' At the time I did not understand it but I did when Malcolm Rae explained it. It is simply a matter of treating the whole person, not just a particular illness. You must treat the mental, spiritual and physical before you can obtain perfect health.

Malcolm Rae then examined me by machine and found that although I had no cancer, I was suffering from cobalt radiation poisoning of the jaw bone, but that the tea was ridding me of that slowly.

Upon our arrival back in Nassau we found thousands of complaints from people who had not received their tea, ordered weeks before. We checked back and found that all had been sent via the Post Office within two days of receiving the order. It seemed as though the powers that be had finally found a way to stop us from helping people. During a period of three months over 10,000 packets of tea disappeared in the post, and we never have found them. The customers, knowing nothing of our problems, started to write some pretty awful letters to us, some even blaming us for their spouse's death.

This of course bothered me to no end, so we kept sending out second orders free, by the thousands. In spite of all our troubles, the letters kept coming in telling of cures for cancer, arthritis, varicose veins, haemorroids, skin problems and much more. Now that the herbs are supplied by one company these problems have been solved.

Along with complaints come pitiful, sad stories – some that have made us weep. One lady sent back the tea, saying, 'My doctor says I have only a month or so to live and he doesn't want me using this stuff.' And another, 'My husband sneaks your tea into the hospital every night in a thermos. The doctor would be furious if he knew what it was but we told him it's brandy. He feels better each day and the doctor thinks it's his doing.' But the saddest case of all is the following. A woman of 35 came to me because she had cancer of the breast. I spoke to her about my case and she became a different person, excited and happy. She visited her doctor that afternoon and he told her that the cancer had spread to her right eye and brain. She said 'What can I do doctor, shall I take herbs, laetrile, shall I pray?' His answer was, 'Don't waste your time on all of that stuff, it's all garbage. Just face it and get your affairs in order.' The lady went home and killed herself that same day.

Please listen to me when I say that *cancer does not mean death*. We usually start dying as soon as we hear that word. We have been brain-washed into thinking it's a killing disease and we are supposed to die from it. The doctor may well insist that you believe him when he tells you how much time you have left. No one knows how long you have got – it's largely up to you. If you believe the doctor then you will die right on time. We have seen this on many occasions. Your life is up to you, so don't believe any doctor who condemns you to die just because he doesn't understand your illness. There are thousands of people I have met who were expected to die of cancer years ago. They all had one thing in common, and that is they were smarter than their doctor. My doctor is so upset that he was wrong about me, that I didn't die as he said I should, that he won't even talk to me now. Believe me, dear fellow sufferer, if there is one person I do not wish ever to talk to again, it's him.

All I am asking you to do is to change your mind about things, and live. God gave you life, and it's up to you to keep it. Eat properly, think properly, and you will soon notice a difference.

An experiment recently in Europe was very interesting. People with cancer were gathered together, and were all asked this question, 'What do you think your cancer looks like, and what do you think of the medicine that you are given to fight it?'

Group A were in accord that their cancer was like a big black rat, very strong and devouring everything, even the medicine.

Group B said that their cancer was a small lump surrounded by white cells (natural immunity), that were gradually eating the cancer away.

Although these people had the same cancer in the same degree, group A died and group B lived. Please think about this. Jesus said that faith can move mountains.

Dr. Fernie has another theory on cancer. He claims that cancer patients all fall into a certain category. He explained it to me this way. A woman of 45 has a husband who now devotes all his time to his business. Her children have left home either to get married or to live elsewhere. She develops breast cancer. Suddenly she is at the top of her husband's list so far as attention goes, and the children come rushing home. Could we get cancer just to get our own way? I know that if we concentrate we can eliminate pain, or make ourselves happy or sad. If Dr. Fernie is right and we unconsciously make ourselves ill, then we can just as easily make ourselves well. Faith can move mountains!

At another clinic only a cancer patient who has passed a test as a positive thinker will be accepted. Also, the only visitors allowed in to see the patients are positive thinkers – ones who will spread hope and life and enthusiasm. It seems to work too.

A clinic in England treats its cancer patients with a steady diet of asparagus tips. This seems to work. Yet another gets good results with massive doses of vitamins A and C, plus six glasses of carrot juice each day.

Another believes that we get cancer because our pancreas is not putting out enough enzymes to eat up the protein in our diet, so they prescribe 30 pancreatic enzymes each day.

One doctor of nutrition has had success fighting cancer with a solution made from poison ivy. One man cured cancer, he assures me, with two tea-spoons of gasoline each day!

Another man with lung cancer refused to go into the hospital for the treadmill of death. He said he would not accept that he had cancer, and it went away. Many say that my tea brings such hope to people who have had all hope taken away, that they believe they will get well as quickly as I – so they do. Faith can move mountains. As soon as we find out that the medical profession isn't the answer, and people are living in spite of phoney death sentences, then we have to choose between many therapies. It seems that everyone who has beaten terminal cancer writes a book about it, and claims to know the secret and the true answer. I am not one of these. I say that seeing that it's your life you are going to save, then take the best from all of them. None of the things they recommend will hurt you, but leave out the gasoline please, there is an oil shortage.

Let's look at it this way. If there are many types of cancers then there could be many types of cure. You must of course purify your blood first. Now then, we are about to take advantage of all the knowledge gained by people who fought for their lives and won. Please remember that most of them were in worse shape than you to begin with. First thing, when that nice little old lady shows up with the coffee, tell her to disappear and take the coffee with her. Don't let her forget the white sugar and cream because you won't be needing those either. Now, if you are in a hospital it may be a little tough because everyone knows it is almost impossible to get well in a hospital. Just be careful of what you eat. Try to get lots of fresh fruit and vegetables, raw if possible. Whole wheat bread only. Eat twenty raw almonds each day. Take five pancreatic enzymes before each meal. Don't eat canned foods, and stay away from salt. Eat twelve ounces of asparagus each day, and if it must be canned use the Jolly Green Giant kind because it has less acid in it. Try to get lots of fresh carrot juice and drink it within an hour of being made. Try to get some laetrile tablets and take four 500mg. tablets each day.

Now I don't want to shock you, but coffee is good for one thing, and one thing only. That is a coffee enema. You laugh, but thousands of ex-cancer patients do this daily and it's simply wonderful for ridding the body of toxins and cleaning the liver. Three cups of strong black coffee in an enema bag, luke warm. Lie on your right side and try to hold it for fifteen minutes, then expel. You will soon find out how much you needed it. You will find it hard to believe all the junk you have been hanging on to all these years. Please don't worry about this becoming habit forming. I know of many people who have had coffee enemas every day for years. As soon as they stop they eliminate naturally again. At one clinic in France they won't let you stay if you refuse to have your regular coffee enema. Here you are already worrying if it's habit forming when just now you were sure you were going to die right away. You see, we've made progress already.

You can drink as much of the herbal tea as you wish. It's God's natural food so it won't harm you and there are no side effects. Even the Russian hockey team drink it daily, just to stay healthy.

One more thing. If you are going to keep on smoking then forget about all of the above. Out of the thousands of terminal patients that I have spoken to during the last three years not one smoker has survived, and it didn't matter what he tried. Once a heavy smoker myself, I can hardly stand to be in the same room as someone who is smoking.

You must quit smoking if you want to live, and if you want to live then you will. Faith can move mountains.

7. A New Life

If you have been subjected to cobalt radiation and/or x-rays then you are suffering a little from radiation poisoning. It's no accident that doctors and nurses disappear behind lead doors while they bombard you with rays.

Here's how to get rid of the ill-effects.

Pour one pound of pure salt purchased from a health food store (not iodized), and one pound of baking soda, into a hot bath and stay in the water for twenty minutes. Immerse the part affected if possible. Do this twice each week for one month. If you have any surgical scars or radiation burns, spread on vitamin E liberally over the affected parts.

Many people I have spoken to have gall stones on top of their other problems. Here

is what a top American nutritionist told me
to do about this, simply and easily without
surgery.

My whole family have done this successfully.

Drink one quart of apple juice daily for
five days. This will soften up the stones to
such an extent that you can squash them in
your fingers.

On the sixth day, skip dinner and at 6
p.m. take a tablespoonful of epsom salts
with water. Repeat at 8 p.m. At 10 p.m.
make a cocktail of four ounces of olive oil
and four ounces of fresh squeezed lemon
juice. Shake vigorously and drink right
down. In the morning you will pass green
stones varying from the size of grains of
sand to some as large as your thumb nail.
You won't feel a thing, but will be amazed
at the results. Thousands have done this
instead of major surgery.

In closing I would like to say that my
heart goes out to you. I don't know you but
I know what you are going through. Thousands are going through the exact same

thing as you right now, so you are not alone.
You have been luckier than the others
though, for you found this book, and now
you know that you don't have to die; you
can live on in health as so many of us are
doing. You can tell of your recovery and so
help others. I didn't start to live until I had
cancer, and I know that it will be the same
for you. Miracles are happening every day
in many places. At the Hans Nieper clinic
in Germany, the Contreras clinic in Mexico;
Dr. Kelly in Washington. Just go and see
for yourself. You will be surprised. Read the
many books at your local health food store,
all about cancer. Cancer is a mystery only
to the medical profession who know nothing
whatsoever about the most important thing
in the world, nutrition. Stay away from
negative people – you don't need their bad
vibrations. Tell them to stay away until you
are better. Start planning on how you will
be spending next year and the year after.
Plan to spread the good word throughout
the country. Cancer no longer means death.

Modern day medicine in North America

spends all of its time treating effects instead of causes. They never find out what causes a swelling, but they treat the swelling. If you cut your finger badly, and then let it get dirty, blood poisoning will set in. After a while a red line will travel up your arm and cause a lump under your armpit. The correct way to treat this is to get rid of the poison and also treat the finger, then the lump will disappear.

Right now it's up to you, completely. Think that you are going to live – like Jason Winters and thousands of others. Watch what you eat. Remember that out of seven years of medical training American doctors have only had six hours on nutrition. You are solely, completely and definitely 100% responsible for yourself. Whatever other people want to do to you, you must always remain captain of your ship.

If you are a cancer patient, I know what you are going through. If in hospital you are surrounded by people who think you are going to die because they don't understand cancer. Red-eyed friends and relatives gather around your bed telling you that everything is going to be fine, even though they don't believe it.

You are there with cancer and your mind runs wild. Every little ache and pain says, 'My God it has spread to my right eye, my left shoulder, my big toe.' Just because you have cancer does not mean that you are immune from all the every-day aches and pains that everyone has to endure. 99 times out of 100 the pain you feel is totally unrelated to cancer. Get that firmly set in your mind. The white cells are eating your cancer, and with a little help from you the tumor may soon be gone.

Getting well again for you will include purifying your body by freeing it of toxins. Fruit, vegetables, fresh juice and the herbal tea will do this, as long as you are not pouring more poison into your body at the same time.

You also need an enema regularly. It comes as a great surprise to many people to learn that Jesus spoke to the Essenes about enemas. As a matter of fact, there is a whole sermon that He gave on the subject of healing in *The Gospel of Peace*.

'Seek therefore a large trailing gourd, having a stalk the length of a man; take out its inwards and fill it with water from the river which the sun has warmed. Hang it upon the branch of a tree, and kneel upon the ground before the angel of water, and suffer the end of the stalk of the trailing gourd to enter your hinder parts, that the water may flow through all your bowels. Afterwards rest kneeling on the ground before the angel of water and pray to the living God that he will forgive you all your past sins, and pray the angel of water that he will free your body from every uncleanness and disease. Then let the water run out from your body, that it may carry away from within it all the unclean and evil-smelling things of Satan ... And this holy baptising by the angel of water is: Rebirth unto the new life.'

Pick up this book and its sequel, *The*

Gospel of the Essenes, and read them carefully. They show that God really does want us all to be healthy – and that is why He gave us instructions that are so explicit. We must pay close attention to this wisdom, remembering that the internal parts of our bodies are perfect places for breeding all types of germs and bacteria, being dark, warm and damp.

Take a positive step; don't think about it, just do it. Buy a bag of fresh fruit. An apple, an orange, a banana and a packet of unblanched almonds or apricot kernels. Go for a walk and as you walk eat the fruit and know that with every bite you are getting enzymes enough to help you. Each step you take will build up your muscles, and the apricot kernels or almonds will give you protein and B17. Already you are doing something sensible to get back to good health. Do this twice a day. You will soon be over the shock and in a better frame of mind. Know with every step you take that another reader in the next town is doing the same thing. We have reports that thousands are doing just this, every day, across the country. Now is the time to get into step with this new army of people. They and you are following others who have already won the fight.

Please believe me when I say that this could be the most important turning point of your life. You have at last stopped your headlong, selfish rush through life, and now you can stand still for a moment, and look around. Those of you who have not noticed the beauty of the world will certainly do so now. Those who were their own god, ignoring their Father in heaven, will find themselves forced to follow God's wisdom in order to survive, and will love Him for every day He gives them. Be humble, assure Him that you will help others from now on, and if you mean it you can live a very long happy life. Today then is the day you start living. God will bless you.

8 The Immune System

The world's leading manufacturer of laetrile (amygdalin), with head offices in Germany, explains cancer this way:

'In spite of numerous costly efforts of medical science, the reason for the uncontrolled division of cancer cells is still unknown. Even a single cell shows a remarkable ability to adapt and survive.

'If its environment is disturbed or changed, the cell will immediately adapt itself.

'This powerful adaptability is comparable to the growing tolerance of insects to pesticides. It is definitely a fact that inflammation or constant stress can lead to cancer. The formation of a cancerous tumor is the defence of the attacked cell to survive.

'The immune system in our body detects and controls the beginning of inflammation. It gives the order to remove or neutralise damaged or destroyed cells.

'But if stress or inflammation continue, for example in skin cancer by over-exposure to the sun, or in cancer of the stomach and intestines by permanent psychological stress, enzymes give orders for cell division in order to bring the body back to its original healthy state.

'The natural survival process begins. But the sick cells confuse the immune system by posing as healthy ones. The result is the gradual reduction of constant orders for cell destruction.

'This weakened immune system can no longer differentiate between a masked, resistant cancer cell and a healthy one. Therefore an uncontrolled division of sick cells takes place.

'The immune system of the cancer patient must be activated to the point where it can once again identify the sick, steadily dividing cancer cells, and kill them. This means that the immune system must be forced into an emergency situation. Many practitioners have been successful by administering mega doses of certain vitamins, vegetable or mineral substances. This brings about an elevation of the immune system where it can once again identify and destroy cancer cells. Unfortunately, unwanted side effects can occur through such over-doses.

'Amygdalin/laetrile/B17 is an extract from bitter almonds or apricot kernels. It is of the utmost importance that only the purest form of this substance is used.

'The atom construction of this substance consists of a cyano group which is very toxic. Only the right, exact procedures in its making will guarantee the ineffectiveness of these toxic substances. Now harmless, the cyan in the laetrile simulates an alarm situation in the cancerous body. Our bodies do not only need vitamins and minerals, but also enzymes. It is therefore of the utmost importance that enough enzymes are administered directly to the bloodstream during the phase of activation.

'Many alternative therapy clinics are administering an intravenous drip solution of enzymes and laetrile at the same time. This is most successful. Clinical tests have brought almost instant relief even to long-suffering cancer victims.

'Also, an insulin-dependent diabetic, for instance, once the pancreas was activated in this manner, showed such progress that insulin injections could be drastically reduced. Rheumatic and gouty pains disappeared.'

This information was sent to me for entry in this book. I have visions of bleary-eyed cancer patients asking, 'What did all that mean?' It means simply this. If your God-given immune system was working properly, you would not have cancer. We now have to start it working. Laetrile will set off an alarm that will wake up your immune system.

EARLY WARNING SIGNS OF CANCER

After talking to over 10,000 cancer victims we found that in every case they had suffered at least three, and often all, of the following danger signals from three to 18 months prior to cancer. There are other warnings which the body may provide, so if in doubt seek medical advice.

1. Weakening of the eyes, necessitating two or three changes of eye glasses in just a few months.

2. Fatigue. You can never get enough rest. You are as tired when you get up in the morning as when you retired at night. You have little or no energy.

3. Nerves. You become easily agitated and quickly fly into a rage. You hurt the ones you love. Self pity overcomes you and you

could easily cry. You become too nervous to go out alone or enter a crowded room.

4. Depression. Life no longer seems worth living. Nothing excites you any more. Morbid thoughts creep into your mind. You quite often become preoccupied with death.

5. A strange tingling, aching sensation deep in your bones. In bed you feel that you must keep changing position, and when you do the aching only goes away for a few minutes.

6. Loss of interest in sexual intercourse.

9 Anxiety

A well-known psychiatrist said, "In the beginning was the word, and the word was anxiety." This pretty well sums up most people's lives. We worry about the endless varieties of hazards, difficulties and disappointments that lay ahead of us.

From the moment we are born, we are surrounded by uncertainties and insecurities. Murphy's Law tells us that life is tough, that few things work out well, and that if a thing can go wrong it usually will. We find out that our idols have feet of clay, that doctors can be wrong, that our favorite movie star is really quite terrible. We are told that God is dead, and there is no one left to fight the F.D.A. No one can stop them putting poisonous flouride in our drinking water, or tons of white sugar in baby food. There is no one powerful enough to say stop, to all the drug ads for high blood pressure, or Valium, Aspirins and Bufferin.

You meet a top reverend (I did), whom in the quiet of his study laughed at the virgin birth and called Billy Graham a charlaton.

Fear is something tangible, and we can usually deal with that. But, anxiety is a very different matter. Anxiety is a state of mind, and is far more lethal. I say lethal because all of these problems eventually manifest themselves in physical illness.

People suffering from anxiety usually do not know which way to turn, so they do nothing. This only increases our anxiety. This, of course, is a mistake.

Growing up is often one long anxiety. "How is my school work? What about the pimples on my face? What job should I choose? Will I be able to keep it? Will people like me?" Then, a few years later, we fall in love and get married. "Will it last? Will he still love me? Who will change first? Who will die first? Will I be able to cope?

No wonder we keep getting ill. With anxiety a person has usually become inbound, an introvert. Serving others is a sure-fire way to become mentally well. Believing in God and keeping busy serving others with kindness and love will usually dispel all your anxieties.

Believing in God is the prime prerequisite because anyone who thinks their life has no meaning, that the world happened by accident, and there is no purpose to anything, has a damn good right to have anxieties. I would suggest that anyone that feels this way is well qualified for a job with the authorities.

Tests have shown that most cancer patients suffer from anxiety prior to the appearance of the tumor. My case was no exception. Months before my tumor, I felt nervous, tense and strangely agitated, even walking into a crowded room bothered me. My right tonsil (site of later cancer) would itch constantly. On going to a doctor, he put me on Valium. This depressed the symptoms and allowed the cancer to grow undetected, until it was almost too late.

Tests also show that most people suffering from mental disorders are simply allergic to certain foods or have a total lack of a necessary chemical or vitamin in their body.

Four Years Later . . .

10 Tibet

The ancient Yogi stepped out of his small hut, high in the Himalayas. In spite of the bitter cold weather and the deep snow, he was clad only in a thin loincloth. His bare feet sunk deep into the snow as he made his way to the small field opposite his hut.

He then sat down in the snow, arranged himself in the lotus position, closed his eyes and began to concentrate. In his mind his spine was a white, hot flame, increasing in size and temperature.

The strangers that had gathered to watch were all, without exception, wearing very thick clothing, including heavy parkas with fur hoods. They were still cold.

The old man did not move a muscle, but

soon it was evident that he was perspiring. Beads of sweat poured down his forehead, arms and chest.

Whispering started among the bystanders. "Could it be, is it possible?" Yes, it was true. The snow around the Yogi had started to melt and trickle away, only to refreeze once outside a six-foot radius.

Wider and wider became the circle around the man. The snow once four inches deep had now gone, and the bare earth could be seen.

Another fifteen minutes found the Yogi in the center of a circle six feet in diameter and completely devoid of snow. Steam arose from this circle, and from the man.

The Yogi then stood up and returned to his hut.

The bystanders walked over to the circle and, taking off their gloves, felt the bare ground with their hands. The heat was like an oven. It soon cooled, however, and the bystanders continued on their way.

Only two were left standing in the circle. Jan looked up at me from under the hood of her parka, and I returned her gaze. No words were spoken as we turned and walked slowly down the mountain trail to the village of Nangchen Japo.

Learning that there is more to life than just existing, more to life than eating, drinking, breathing and working has brought to my life renewed enthusiasm and vitality.

To find myself standing on a mountain in Tibet, watching the ancient Yogi definitely was exciting, and a far cry from selling refrigerators back in Canada.

It came about this way: One morning, while relaxing in my study in the sixteenth century cottage that we now call home, on the south coast of England, I received a very strange letter postmarked China.

It was from a Buddhist group that had been using the herbal tea for over one year. They were excited about it and invited me to visit with them as their guest. All I had to do was to get there.

Jan, my wife, was excited about this also, for to get a letter of praise from far-off China, a country wise in the use of herbs for thousands of years, was praise indeed.

Although the invitation was just for me, I

decided to take my dear wife along on a kind of holiday. It had been raining steadily in our county for about two weeks.

We arrived at the Hilton Hotel in Hong Kong, right on the island, a place so full of sights, sounds and smells that it boggles the mind. I received word that I would be met the following morning by a Buddhist monk at the Shangri La Hotel in Kowloon, and that "the invitation" was just for me. My wife took this very well, and I left her some money for shopping and the next day I took the ferry to the pier on the Kowloon side.

The man that met me was not dressed in bright saffran, as I had expected, but in a darker robe. He appeared to be at least one hundred years old, with wrinkled face and glittering, healthy eyes full of life. It was like walking with a child, for I am almost six foot five inches tall, and he was slightly under five feet. He walked fast and was obviously excited, and his English was quite good.

He explained that we must take a train towards Guangchou and then disembark and walk two and a half miles. He did not tell me that it would be a very steep, uphill walk all the way.

Arriving at the temple tired, hot and out of breath, I was shown to a room with only a table, one chair and a slab of rock on which to sleep. On the table was a pitcher full of water and a bowl to wash in. A drone of male singers echoed through the myriads of rooms and hallways and into my room. As I washed a chill came over me suddenly as I remembered where I was, alone, thousands of miles away from home in an atmosphere so totally foreign to me.

Another very old man came into the room carrying a bowl of rice with some kind of vegetable mixed with it, and a bowl of brown drink. I tasted it carefully and behold, it was my herbal tea.

Going into the main hall later that day, I noticed that only men were to be seen, and that these men were all of great age. The eldest was by far the wisest, and although very short and thin, he looked as though he was amazingly healthy. His voice was high and melodic, and he spoke English in flowery tones. He greeted me and shivers ran down my back, and for some unknown reason, the hair on the back of my neck stood on end. "Did you know, Mr. Jason, that you are 49 years younger than the youngest man at this temple? You are now 51 years of age, are you not?" He smiled at my surprise. "Mr. Jason, I am now 139 years of age." When I asked him to what he attributed his longevity, he answered thus, "You in the Western World are led to believe that you are born, must go to school, graduate, enter college, get a 'good' job, work under high pressure, and at 65 you retire and prepare to die. You have all been brainwashed by very unhealthy teachings from very unhealthy people. You have a complete lack of understanding of life and death. A man does not get wise until he is 65. He has not absorbed everything he can until 80. He is 100 years of age before he can introduce into his daily life this wisdom and experience. He knows instinctively that he is what he thinks, as well as what he eats at this age. The next 40 years of his life are easy and happy. He has no fears of life, death or illness. Apart from an accident, he must remain healthy and productive because he eats and thinks properly. He has the right attitude

91

towards everything. You in the West expect to die early, so you do. You really make no connection between yourselves and God. Of course, you are a part of God, and with this understanding only then do you realize that you do what you think you will do. Westerners expect to become ill periodically, so they do. They expect to die early, so they do.

"Try expecting to live long and be healthy. Combine this with the wisdom of living and you will do and become whatever you want. Nothing can stop you."

I asked him about the herbal tea and he told me that the monks use it constantly. It's part of the settling of the mind and purifying of the body that we need in order that we may direct our thinking and our lives in the right direction.

I had noticed that the whole time I was there in the monastery that the aged monks would take out a small package of powder and place some on their tongues. At last I ventured to ask about this, and the answer was in one of the most beautiful stories that I have ever heard.

It seems that when Bayan of a Thousand

Eyes came out of Mongolia leading his great army, he brought with him hundreds of weak and wounded from continuous battles fought across the continent. After ravaging Peking, they proceeded onto the ancient city of Xian. Once there, the troops were amazed at the amount of very old, but agile and active people living in that town. They soon found that all the residents of the that town took a special herb mixture every day without fail. Babies were fed this soon after they became three months of age. A small pinch of the herbs would be placed on their tongues.

The soldiers also found that this mixture was used only once each day after the morning meal, never at any other time. The local physicians started giving this to the weak and wounded soldiers, who soon found their strength returning very quickly. But something else was happening, too. They also found that they felt better than ever before in their entire lives. Every soldier given this formula, according to legend, recovered. Legend also tells us that they all lived to a ripe old age.

The ancient gentleman leaned towards me and continued, "This herb mixture allows men to enjoy sexual relations over the age of one hundred, and keeps their bodies trim, virile and strong, their minds active and alert. It also allows women to remain beautiful, feminine, and, above all, content into a very old age. That is why we like *your* formula so much, Mr. Jason, for it is very compatible with what we already are taking, although it serves a different purpose entirely."

He then suggested that we visit Tibet, "The Rooftop of the World," to find even more intriguing insights into the secrets of long life and good health. That is why Jan and I visited the Yoga and were privileged to watch that astounding display.

Finally we come to Dr. Forbes Ross, whom published his revolutionary book in London in 1912.

This man made quite a discovery. To all of his patients he would prescribe 60 grains of citrate of potash in distilled water. He realized that even then people desperately needed potassium to remain healthy. He discovered that in all of his years in practice he never had one patient come down with cancer. Also, the new patients that came to him with cancer were all well soon after taking the potash regularly.

We today suffer from potassium starvation, and it is interesting to note that if cancer is a "germ" disease, it has recently been found that potassium is nature's supreme antiseptic.

Interestingly enough, The National Enquirer, March 1983 issue claims that Karen Carpenter's death was caused by very low potassium level due to her other problems with anorexia nervosa. I quote, "Low potassium levels causes irregular heartbeats which can lead to heart failure.

Potassium is needed as a daily supplement, so I have added it to the Jason Winters **"Take It For Health"** list that is so popular in Europe.

11 Herbal Legacies

An eagle sat on his perch, high on the mountain, and gazed at the valley below. It was moving as though the whole earth was alive. It was in reality Buffalo by the millions, all heading south for the winter.

A lone camp fire raised smoke down by a small creek, and whenever a buffalo came too close he would be felled by many arrows shot by the Indian braves in hiding. At the same times the squaws and maidens would be gathering herbs and preparing for the evening meal around the campfire. One herb they would pick was well known for treating swollen joints and fevers, another was for innerstrength and wellbeing. These valuable herbs would be mixed with almost everything the women prepared.

This scene took place centuries before the first Spanish explorer tracked his way across the great American Southwest. Yet the women were well aware that they were practicing preventative medicine and also curing many ills.

There are few eagles left today, and hardly any buffalo. The eagle now flies through polluted air, and drinks from heavily polluted rivers. But the knowledge of those ancient indian women live on, and it is this knowledge and not modern science that will lead the few who will listen through to the new age in good health and safety.

At the same time that the eagle watched the great buffalo migration another migration was taking place in an unheard of land half way around the world.

Long before the Chinese were invaded from the north, and long before the cities of Canton and Peking had its first settlers, China was ruled by the capitol city of Xian. The migration taking place here was to prove most important to the healers of all China, India and Tibet.

Powerful holy men, with a vast knowledge of herbal remedies would travel far and wide to cities and villages, just for the honor of giving talks in the market places, imparting knowledge to the poor and ailing on how to regain abundant health and happiness.

Some of these travelling teachers found themselves in a far off high country that would one day be called Tibet. They were excited to find that the rarified air, due to the extreme elevation, was conducive to clear thinking and spiritual uplifting that allowed them a closer contact with God.

Because of this, many villages would spring up with its own monastery, filled with monks or holy men. Because they believed in reincarnation, (many lives) and the law of karma, (cause and effect) they were very kind and gentle to each other. Each morning the villagers would lay at the gates of the monasteries baskets of medicinal herbs, which were used by the holy men daily.

Hundreds of years later, in 2838 B.C. the Chinese emporer SHENG NOONG would compile the worlds first list of these herbs, and their uses. He mentioned 365 herbs in all.

Long before the Mayflower reached America, and long before Ponce de Leon arrived in Florida looking for his fountain of youth, the viking sailed into natural harbours all up and down the coast of North and South America, from Nova Scotia to Rio.

In South America they found the great rain forests, and were overcome by the extreme dampness, the mildew and the rot that prevailed. Everything was covered with moss, fungus and insects. Everything that is except a certain type of tree that stood tall, strong and unblemished. No decay or fungus had touched this tree. No insects made their home in its bark. In this unhealthy climate this tree survived and was every bit as beautiful as the trees they were used to in far off Norway and Sweden.

The Vikings learned much from the natives of South America, and when at last they were to turn their ships homeward, it was not gold and silver they would be taking back, but bark, bark that would bring a higher price than gold in their own land. For the voyagers had learned that since time immemorial, this bark, made into a liquid would successfully fight off all diseases and would greatly speed up the healing of accident victims. Medical scientists in South America have recently found that this bark contains a very powerful anti biotic. It is now famous world wide, (except in America) and is proving invaluable to many clinics and hospitals.

It makes no difference what ancient culture we wish to discuss, the fact remains that they knew something that we do not. They were closer to nature and closer to GOD. Their knowledge grew over thousands of years of trial and error, until at last they knew the values of plants and herbs.

Considering the billions of dollars spent by modern science the results prove that they have failed miserably. But they have succeeded in one respect!! They have certainly managed to keep the ancient knowledge written about here a secret in North America, where sickness and medication are the most expensive in the world.

12 The Thymus

For many years doctors thought that the thymus gland was just something that helped a child grow, and once an adult, then it served no purpose. The thymus lies just beneath the upper breastbone, in the middle of the chest. They thought that once the person became an adult, the gland should shrivel.

As a matter of fact, as recently as the early nineteen fifties, if doctors came across a patient with a large (healthy) thymus they would give him cobalt radiation to try to reduce its size. Many brilliant doctors now know that the thymus is the seat of a persons immune system, and the only reason it grows smaller in most adults in America is because of stress and worry. Dr. John Diamond, in his new book, "YOUR BODY DOESN'T LIE" has proven that you can tell a persons life force through testing the thymus. Beautiful thoughts, paintings, music make the thymus strong, negative thoughts, ugly sights, and rock and roll music drastically weakens the thymus and therefore your life force almost instantly.

If you are jealous, vindictive, full of hatred, closed minded then your thymus shrivels and you become weak. If a Dr. tells you you're terminal, your body tests weak immediately. Just being with a negative person for a little while will leave you feeling weak and exhausted, while the negative person leaves feeling a little stronger.

Dr. Diamond says that he had never seen a sick person that did not have an underactive thymus. He believes that thymus weakness or underactivity is the cause of all illness.

Whether athiests like this or not, while in church, or praying, or helping some unfortunate person, your life force strengthens and your thymus becomes healthier.

One thing Diamond mentions is that if you have a group of people in a room, and suddenly someone lights up a smoke, within twenty minutes every person in that room will have the same level of nicotene in their blood. A frightening thought.

A sad plight in North America are the elderly. They are constantly told by their doctors, "well, you can expect to be ill at your age" thereby sapping them continually of life force. Add to this the fact that we have been brainwashed into thinking that anyone of seventy years is old, (nothing could be further from the truth) and then the fact that if they do get ill their whole live savings goes immediately to the doctor and hospital, so that even if they recover from this whole negative attitude they have been put under, all they have to look forward to is a meagre old age pension, where they can't even afford the proper nutritious food. As we are all only too aware, junk food is cheap, but nutritious food is almost out of reach for all of us. I wonder if anyone will ever do something about this tragedy. After living in the east I feel that our elderly are dying thirty years before their time, just because they have been told that it is expected. Because of this, I agree with Dr. Mendelsohn M.D. when he states that hospitals are very dangerous places to go. Not only are they rampant with disease but the negative atmosphere literally destroys the life force of most people, let alone the elderly.

After giving the formula of TRIBALENE to a health food manufacturer I thought I would be free of the health food business. But then I was told about Perisel, and I felt that everyone should know about this mixture at once. Both of these products are available freely, (but beware of useless imitations). After Perisel I was sure that I could get out of the health food formulas, but alas, that is not so. Now there is **Xian.**

This is my final formula but it is probably the most important. It consists of herbs that will reactivate the thymus, and you have just read how desperately we all need this. I call this formula Xian, after the great Chinese capitol that was using herbs for healing thousands of years ago.

It is hard to believe that they knew about the thymus, the seat of life, and the life energy way back then. I am certainly very happy to make this my biggest and last contribution to my many friends around the world. Xian is destined, I have been assured, to be used widely by all people whom wish to remain healthy and in good frame of mind.

Peggy Mason is a spiritual writer living in Tunbridge Wells England. She is highly psychic and has helped many around the world whom just seem out of step with todays world. One of her peeves is cruelty to animals. She claims that we do not get away with anything in this life, especially when we are cruel to defenseless animals. Today, for instance, chickens are raised, force fed, in factories specializing in mass production. They are kept all their life in a small cage the same size as their body. No room to move at all, their head is fitted through a small hole in the cage, and they cannot withdraw it, ever! They cannot run, move, scratch or do anything but stand there, all of their lives. This pitiful, desperate, anxious, helpless, unhappy state causes· poisons and toxins to course throughout the chickens body. To eat such a bird simply transfers all that poison to the consumer. And we wonder why we get sick.

Mason also found that unnecessary operations on animals, done simply for practice and fun, have a direct effect on the perpetrator. She was horrified to find at one clinic, dogs living in utter terror, because they had been operated on and now had an extra head grafted on. In spite of the absolute cruelty shown them by man, the dog would still look at a stranger visiting and, with head hung low would try to wag its tail.

Fortunately, these godless experimentors are not happy. According to research, although they somehow can justify this obscene occupation in their own godless minds, they do suffer far more illnesses than the average person. Cancer and heart disease strikes them at a far greater rate. That is what is meant by "As you sow, so shall you reap."

Recently a doctor was so proud of himself while on T.V. He explained that weeks before he had forced a white mouse into a tiny test tube and had sealed the end. A tiny hole was in one end so that the mouse could breath. He showed this on T.V. The mouse, unable to move backwards or forwards could only in desperation turn over and over in a futile attempt to escape. The doctor was trying once again to prove that stress causes cancer. This has been proven hundreds of times already!

I was happy to note that the doctor had a serious case of sanpaku which proved that his smiling face belied his true feelings, and could not hide his physical illness.

Now you may think that all this fuss over a mouse or chicken is ridiculous, but I say to you that just because an animal is helpless and can't talk doesn't mean that it has no feelings. It suffers just as much as would you under the same conditions. Participating in this type of experiment, or knowing about it yet doing nothing to stop it causes a weakening of your life force and will eventually cause the same suffering in your own body, to an equal extent.

Cruelty is not conducive to good health. We can't get away with a thing in this life. We don't need a judge and jury to convict us, we do it ourselves. That is what God meant when he said "Judge not" for we need not judge and sentence others, everyone, no matter how insensitive a person is, sentences themselves.

If you are sure you are going to die, then your thymus will shrivel and you will die. If you are sure, and have faith that you are going to live, then your thymus will expand and start your immune system working at a fast pace, and if you eat nutritiously you will recover.

The whole of this book has been devoted to the story of one mans' pursuit of life and of the desperation forced upon him by the death sentence passed by his medical advisors.

It has portrayed step by step the long march back to eventual triumph using Gods' abundant gifts of nature to put to flight a disease considered by much of the western medical World as incurable.

13 Guides to Good Health

The secret of Jason Winters' success lies wrapped within the mists of antiquity but it would be wrong to assume the only valuable aid to abundant good health comes from ancient times.

The story of GEROVITAL, the "B" Complex formula developed by Professor Dr. Ana Aslan of Romania, is without doubt tremendously impressive. As a beneficial remedy against the degenerative diseases of old age and maladies of the central nervous system this product (often foreshortened GH3) has a history stretching back 30 years — in more than 70 progressive countries — and an estimated usage by upwards of one hundred million people that cannot possibly be ignored. Bearing in mind safety and non-addictive qualities of GH3 it can only be regarded as a most powerful and signifigant companion to TRI-BALENE and XIAN for both remedial and preventative regimes.

For those interested in learning more of this wonderfull product we suggest you contact:

GOOD HEALTH ASSOCIATES INC.
PO BOX 14785
LENEXA,
KANSAS
U.S.A.

GHA INC supplies only top quality GH3 (brand name ASLAN PLUS) and it is important our readers keep well away from the many suspect copies currently available, most of which are totally ineffective and some of which are even harmfull.

Since Ruth Montgomeries new best selling book "Threshold to Tomorrow" became available in every book store, Jason Winters has been deluged with mail each day. (The first chapter of Montgomeries book is dedicated to Jason Winters)

All the letters ask him the same general questions; How should I live?

To expedite matters, Jason answers these questions by telling you what he does daily to maintain perfect health;

Eat 20 Raw unblanched almonds daily,

Take 3 Tribalene capsule, one before each meal.

Take 3 Perisel capsules each morning after breakfast, plus 3 Potassium tablets.

Eat some asparagus daily, as it comes from the can.

Two heaping tablespoonfuls of Brewers yeast in a glass of orange juice each afternoon.

Take 3 XIAN tablets daily to assist the thymus and life force.

Have a sauna or jacuzzi daily (perspire)

Eliminate properly every day. Take one enema each week. High colonic each month.

Have complete faith that you shall live to be one hundred years old. Think good thoughts and expect the very best for yourself.

Stay well away from negative people and people that drain you of your strength.

Listen to good classical or symphony music. Try to watch only pleasant things on television, and read good books, including poetry. They calm your mind.

You are a part of God, and HE loves you very much. You can never be alone, there is nothing that can't be corrected, no one that can't be saved. You can expect the best because you are the best.

A WORD ABOUT DOCTORS

When I wrote my first book, entitled *"Killing Cancer,"* I was pretty discouraged about doctors in general. I guess I had the misfortune of having atheistic, uncaring doctors and so had tarnished them all with the same brush.

During my hundreds of radio and T.V. shows, however, I am very pleased to say that I have discovered many dozens of medical men and women who do, in fact, care greatly about their patients. Some have even admitted to me that they pray sincerely for God's help before even attempting an operation.

Many have said that nutrition is the most vital treatment in all diseases. Even in the case of accidents, they say, proper nutrition is responsible for fast recovery. I am so glad to learn that there are so many caring doctors out there. It should make us all feel so much safer.

As a final word I would like to say that people like myself can tell you about things such as Tribalene and Perisel® which I am sure will cut down your visits to doctors greatly. However, if you should need a doctor look for one carefully. Make sure he believes in a power greater than the A.M.A. Even then . . . always get a second opinion.

The Truth About Perisel.®

"The continuing story of Jason Winters"

BY BENJAMIN ROTH SMYTHE

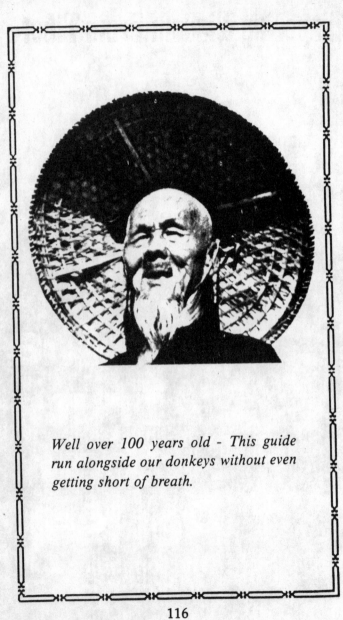

Well over 100 years old - This guide run alongside our donkeys without even getting short of breath.

This is a Story of Four
Very Important Things:

1. SELENIUM T

2. GOTU KOLA

3. TIBETAN SPICE

4. YOUR BLOOD

Carefully mixing Selenium T Special
Spice and Gotu Kola together for the
first time gives us a breakthrough which
we call Perisel®.

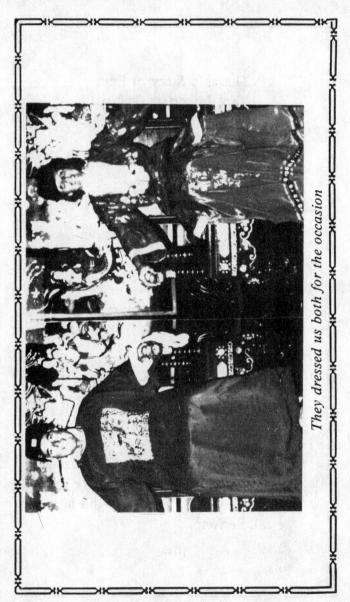

They dressed us both for the occasion

Since arriving in Tibet I have been lightheaded. I am not sure whether is is due to the altitude or rather to the great amount of ancient wisdom given to me by my companion. It was from him, a man well over one hundred years of age, that I learned how to eat, think, and be content.

It seemed strange indeed that an ex terminal cancer patient like me should have to leave America, the scientific leader of the world, and go to far off Tibet to learn something as simple as "How To Live."

I could not help thinking that maybe we are the backward ones. I am curious to find out why it is that an old man, living in a small village in Tibet can tell me things that doctors, scientists and highly intelligent men in America are just now discovering, and at a cost of billions of dollars. A person can return from Tibet with specific information on how to prevent and sometimes cure many of man's ills through herbs and diet secrets that have been tried and tested in Tibet for five thousand years.

Some enthusiasts return to America ready to start right in helping people, only to be told a most definite "No" by one agency or another. It seems that a white coated egg-head must tie up the product for five years before he says it's ok. Something used for five thousand years must now be tested by "one of us".

I am sure that many of us believe that God placed protection and cures for all man's ills right in or on the ground. All the herbs, minerals and vitamins are there, if we only knew which ones were which.

Many countries could help us in this respect. China for one has many thousands of herbalists that have been making people well for years.

Somehow, our medical men and women are off on a tangent of their own, and could not possibly ask assistance from any other than a medical man with the same training as themselves.

Can we really expect more from our medical people? Out of the many years of medical training that they receive, they get about one seven-hour course on nutrition. It should be the other way around.

Growing up in the West is not easy. There is no one to tell us how to eat, think, live. Anyone with the knowledge to help is frowned upon and discouraged. We certainly have a long way to go. If you don't think so then try going on a radio talk-back show as a guest, and talk about a herb that can help sick people. Every doctor within fifty miles will call in and attack you as if you were the devil himself.

Because of this attitude, many truths are kept hidden. I think one of these truths concerns *Selenium T.*

The ancient Tibetan and his friends and family eat a high selenium diet, and they just radiate health. It was because of his certainty about this mineral that I started looking into the research done on this element in the West. I think the results have been astounding, and certainly warrant the writing of this little book.

Selenium T, it could be just what

you have been looking for.

In my travels around the world, I discovered one very important fact. Every group of people that have a low intake of Selenium T suffer fatigue, depression, distressing menopause pains, and more susceptibility to all degenerative diseases, including cancer.

There is a direct relationship between highly civilized countries' processed foods, junk food and lack of selenium.

Selenium is an active mineral that is desperately needed in our bodies, for it is a wonderful antioxident. It has been shown to prevent or at least slow down the aging process. Also it has become famous in some clinics for slowing down hardening of the arteries. Males appear to need Selenium T even more than women. In the male, 50% of their body's supply concentrates in the testicles and the seminal ducts adjacent to the prostrate gland. Also, much selenium is lost in the semen.

"The levels of selenium in the blood of people in various cities has been found to bear a direct relationship to cancer mortality."* The higher the levels of selenium, the lower the cancer death rate and visa versa.

Quoted from the *Vitamin Bible*,
Earl Mindell, Author.

FACTS AND ACTUAL TESTS

Because of a report given by Schwarz and Foltz, and encouraged by the same, Hopkins and Majaj showed that administration of selenium to children in Jordan with Washiorkor stimulated body growth and reticulocyte formation.

Burke reported finding in children from Guatemala with the same ailment, that although they did not respond to a nutritional supplement diet, when selenium was added to the diet, the health of the children improved, and the concentration of selenium in their blood increased to control levels. These finds were confirmed by Levine and Olson.

In English this means simply that children in Jordan and also in Guatemala that were suffering a disease called Washiorkor were cured when selenium was added to their diet. Other diseases also responded when selenium was administered in small doses.

Peridontal Disease is a major health problem in New England, a low selenium area, and has been reported to be associated with selenium deficiency in the sheep and cattle of New Zealand.

Sudden Infant Death Syndrome

The studies of researcher Money suggests that sudden death in human infants may result from the combined deficiencies of Vitamin E and selenium in cow's milk formulas. During the first month of life, breast fed infants received more than ten times the Vitamin E and more than twice the selenium than that of infants fed cow's milk formulas.

Cardiovascular Disease

Researcher Frost compared maps of early heart mortality and cardiovascular related deaths for different areas of the United States and demonstrated an inverse relationship between ambient selenium levels and the death pattern.

Marjanan and Soni, who previously thought that manganese deficiency might underlie the very high cardiac and cancer mortality rate in Finland, have now adopted the view that selenium deficiency, prevalent all over Finland, may be the main contributor.

Lesions of selenium deficiency in rats and sheep have been associated with vascular abnormalities. Demonstrations of the role of selenium in maintenance of membranes may also suggest a function within the vascular system.

Cancer

Investigation of the direct relationship of selenium to human cancer has been limited to demographic studies and to comparisons of levels of selenium in the blood of patients with or without malignancies, Chu and Davidson listed selenium compounds among potential antitumor agents. In addition, Shamberger and Rudolph and Shamberger et al., associated protection from cocarcinogenesis with antioxidents (Vitamin E, selenium, etc.) and food preservation. Harr et al. reported that concentration of dietary selenium delayed or prevented the induction of cancer by N-2-fluorenylacetamide (FAA). The effective concentration of dietary selenium in the torula feed in this experiment was the addition of 100-500ng/g of feed.

On the average, the blood of cancer patients was reported to contain less selenium than the blood of other patients. However, the blood of patients with some forms of cancer showed normal levels of selenium.

Mammary adenocarcinomas induced by FAA in selenium depleted rats were more invasive than those induced in rats fed selenium supplemented foods.

Above from the National Research Council.

Reproductive System

When it comes to nutritional deficiencies, it seems to be the reproductive organs that suffer most. It is only fair to say that an excess of certain elements can cause just as much trouble in this area.

Selenium has done much to explain the distribution of this element in the reproductive system. This could mean that selenium has specific roles in the reproduction systems of male, female and developing offspring.

Kar and co-workers, and later others, found that the testicular damage induced by cadmium salts could be prevented by the administration of selenium dioxide.

It is the belief of many researchers that selenium transports cadmium away from vulnerable sites to other locus within the testes where it is innocuous.

Muth et al. finds that administering selenium to pregnant ewes prevents myopathy in developing lambs. This has since been confirmed by many investigators.

It has also been confirmed through research that selenium does, in fact, pass from the pregnant mother to the unborn child.

Although selenium is present in cow's milk, human milk contains selenium in concentrations twice as high.

Because of the large amount of mercury used today by both industry and agriculture, the amount of selenium reaching the fetus might be diminished and thereby bring about a state of selenium deficiency in the child. Thus the advantage of breastfeeding.

Deficiency in selenium definitely

affects the general health. Rats fed a selenium deficient diet over a few generations showed adverse effects on reproduction.

The female offspring failed to reproduce when mated with normal males. The male offspring had defects in their sperm — it was immotile (incapable of spontanious movement).

In further studies on piglets from selenium starved sows, it was shown that lesions appeared first in the connective tissue and capillaries.

Sprinkler found that rats starved of selenium suffered a thickening and degeneration in tissues such as the cardiac muscle, testes, and retina. Because of this, researchers Sweeny and Brown concluded that selenium deficiency causes primary damage to the vasculature (blood channels) and also had a bad effect on the membranes.

Selenium was found to be an anti-inflammatory mineral, which resulted in selenium tocopheral treatments for chronic lameness in dogs.

Researcher Money found that over forty species of mammals and birds cannot tolerate selenium deficiency. It is all important in their lives.

Selenium deficiency became an agricultural problem after World War Two because of the changes in animal nutrition. To deal with this the Food and Drug Administration approved the use of selenium as a food additive.

Although the importance of selenium in the case of animals is well known, little is known about its role in human beings. Reports from some laboratories indicate that selenium may have anticarcinogenic properties. Also, selenium has been found to have some inhibitory effect on the development of tumors in rodents injected with carcinogens.

Selenium is used as an anti-dandruff preparation and also as an anti-fungal agent in Tinea Versicolor.

Alternative therapy clinics around the world are using selenium in small doses to try to counteract degenerative diseases, and great promise is being shown.

GOTU KOLA

"REVITALIZE YOUR SEX LIFE"

GOTU KOLA
The Second Ingredient

Gotu Kola has been used in many countries around the world, where they claim benefits such as relieving mental fatigue, age spots, aging, brain problems, lack of energy, endurance, high blood pressure, poor memory, pituitary problems, senility, menopause and loss of vitality.

REVITALIZES YOUR SEX DRIVE

This herb, mixed with the others mentioned, restores sexual desire and activity within just a few weeks. This approach is natural, with no harmful hormone injections or tablets. Doctors will not give hormones to people with cancer, or to those susceptible to cancer. If ancient Tibetans enjoy sex in their nineties and older, then why should we not be able to do the same?

It seems that Gotu Kola strengthens the mind, gives one the ability to cope with life and its stresses. Many say it gives renewed confidence and zest for life.

Many alternative clinics around the world are using this herb with success. Once, carried from India on the backs of mules, this herb is now grown very successfully in Tibet, and is used both in Tibet and India for mental problems of all kinds. Combined with the vital spice from Tibet, we have Perisel.

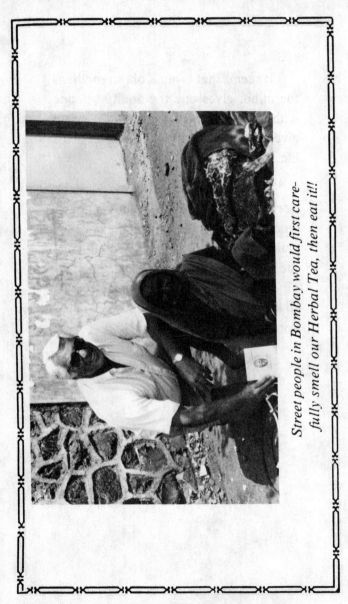

Street people in Bombay would first care-fully smell our Herbal Tea, then eat it!!

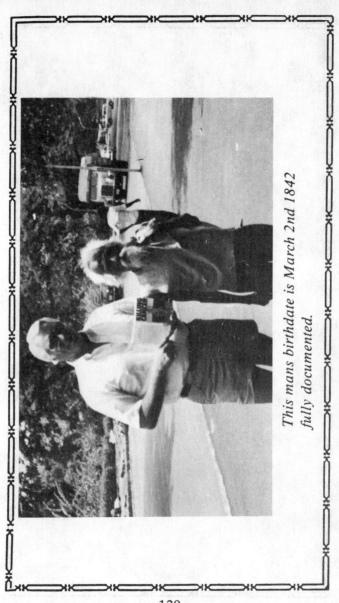

*This mans birthdate is March 2nd 1842
fully documented.*

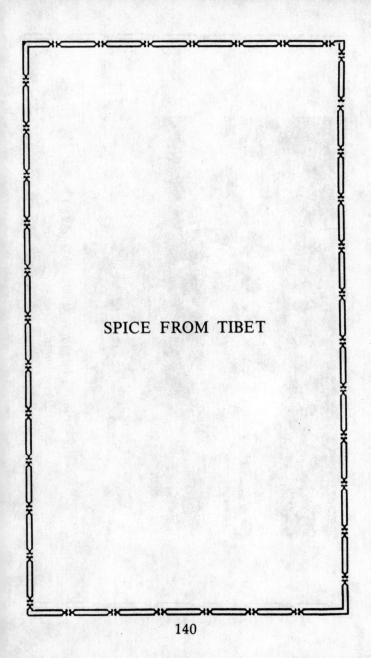

SPICE FROM TIBET

Hundreds of years ago, a great army pushed its way across Mongolia, China and Tibet, raping and pillaging every foot of the way. In spite of confiscating all the poor farmers' crops, the soldiers were quite often very hungry and would have perished in the winter blizzards if it were not for the secrets passed down to them for thousands of years. One great secret was SPICE. Not just an ordinary Spice, but one to give strength, purity and stamina. At night, while the weary soldiers slept the "Physicians and Medics", who were really herbalists, would scour the countryside looking for healing herbs.

The spice we call TIBETAN SPICE was really a find, for this particular herb was the one they knew would put all the solders who were feeling poorly, back into shape quickly.

It seems that even in those days there was such a thing as 'sick call', which was held early in the morning before starting out on another long day's travel.

The Herbalists were highly thought of and were carried all day between two horses. They slept mostly, and then at night, with the aid of large flaming torches, they foraged for herbs.

So highly thought of were these herbalist-physicians, that during battle they were kept well to the rear in both luxury and safety.

Not only was it their job to treat wounds and help the fighting soldiers recover quickly, but they were also charged with keeping the whole army healthy. By this I mean that they had to practice PREVENTIVE MEDI-CINE. If too many soldiers came down with sickness other than wounds obtained on the battlefield, they would be severely reprimanded.

You see, in those days a physician's main job was to teach the soldiers how to keep well. What a wonderful way to look at the medical profession. To keep people well. To teach them how to Eat, Think and Live correctly.

Even in those days they knew that preventing an illness was better than treating one, and so the spice mentioned here was treasured by all. This knowledge has been passed down to us today.

Here is what modern researchers say about this particular SPICE.

"It is helpful if you want to burn the candle at both ends." This miracle medicinal herb from early times reputedly cured a thousand ills and prevented the onslaught of old age. Greek doctors of old regarded this herbal spice as a sacred herb. Dioscorides used it as a remedy: sore throats, snake bite, tuberculosis, kidney troubles, ulcers, arthritis, and lack of ambition and drive, among other things.

An old Arab proverb states, "How can a man die, with this spice available to him?"

Properly prepared it does away with decay, is good for the memory, makes a person stronger and prevents spiritual depression. "It makes the life force strong until the end," states another authority. This means that there is no degeneration of faculties during old age.

In PERISEL®, it gives the other two ingredients a definite and powerful boost that cannot be denied. Grown in America, this spice can only be as good as the nutrients in the earth.

If the correct nutrients are missing, then the herb or vegetable has no good effect on the body. We in America, however, are content with growing food that looks good but in reality has no food value. We also shower the earth with poisons and chemicals to make plants grow quickly and larger than normal. Then quite often we polish the food with wax that is definitely detrimental to a person's health.

We, in actuality, end up eating something that looks great but is an almost "dead food" in our bodies.

Tibetan spice is carefully grown. It is cultivated in naturally rich soil, containing all the ingredients that GOD intended which are so necessary to our good health.

THE BLOOD

LIFE IS IN THE BLOOD

The Mysterious Essence

For many thousands of years, since man began to question his place in the universe and his relationship to life itself, blood, the flowing essence of life, has played an important role in his search for meaning, and whole mythologies have grown around it. The scriptures of the world are filled with references to blood as the bearer of life. Physiologically it carries a continuous supply of nutrients and oxygen to all parts of the body and removes debris and waste gases and other impurities. According to the Vedic teachings the life-principle anchored in the heart of man is able to blend with the blood and thus carry the life-force (or Prana) to all areas of the organism; Prana is the name given to those energizing forces which flow from the sun. The heart, working in conjunction with the spleen, distributes these solar energies to vitalize the physical form.

The relationship between blood and life is evident. Death comes as blood leaves the body. The monthly flow of menstrual blood in the human female temporarily ceases its cyclic flow as a new life in the form of a child begins to make its appearance. Blood is, in a sense, the essence of life; and out of this, no doubt, grew the belief that the power to revitalize and regenerate lies in blood sacrifice.

The Greeks said that spirits gathered at sacrifices in order to absorb the life forces of the spilled blood. Such is the power present in shed blood, wrote Paracelsus, that its emanations provide enough matter to form a visible body for a discarnate entity.

Many thousands of years ago people ceremonially coated the bodies of their dead with a red mineral pigment called Haematite. Haematite is a Greek word meaning 'Blood-Stone', and its use in burial was universal. Graves between 20,000 and 45,000 years old, as far apart as Siberia, France, Bavaria, Wales and South Africa, all show clear evidence of an ancient belief in life forces contained in Blood-Stone. Both African and Australian tribesmen relate the legend of the Mother Goddess of the Earth whose blood soaked into the soil to form a great deposit of Haematite. Even today, Blood-Stone is used for healing purposes to stop bleeding of the lungs and uterus, as an antidote to snakebite, and to clear bloodshot eyes. It is also used as a cosmetic in Africa for ritual purposes, and similar uses were made of it by the native.

The use of blood in religious ritual has been replaced in the modern world by substitute elements. This is symbolized most clearly in the Eucharist, where the initiate partakes of the body of Christ through the wafer and of the blood of Christ through the wine, consecrated beforehand by appropriate rituals and prayer.

The Rosicrucian Max Heindel wrote that the soul controls the dense physical body by way of the blood which is its particular vehicle. Empedocles in 480 B.C. stated that 'Blood is Life', and Goethe had Faust say that man's blood is a liquid fire. Steiner spoke of the blood as containing a record of the life of the individual, registering every thought and emotion; life being transmitted from the ethers through breath to the lungs and there making its impress on the blood. All mystics agree with Jacob Boehme that the spirit of God moves in the blood of man, and everyone is familiar with the Christian phrase, 'Saved by the Blood of Christ'. There are, of course, many interpretations of this, and some recognize that it can mean the reorganization of the energies within the individual as the Christ comes to birth within him.

Buddhist texts outline techniques for determining the nature of another's thoughts through the color of his or her heart-blood: such cognition is produced by developing the power of clairvoiance in order to see the heart-blood. If the person has happy thoughts then the colors seen are red, like the ripe banyan fruit; if sad thoughts, then the color is black; and if the thoughts are predominantly neutral, the heart-blood appears to have the color of clear sesamum oil.

A WORD OF WARNING

Did you know that the F.D.A. has no jurisdiction over the tobacco companies, yet I feel that tobacco kills more people every day than all the wars in history.

Also, tobacco companies are subsidized by the government. What a fantastic and remarkable thing to be taking place in a country such as America, where we pride ourselves on a "government for the people."

People that smoke have no way of knowing that not only does their breath smell terrible, but also their hair, their clothes, their car, their house and their furniture.

The glamour of smoking soon leaves when at last they find themselves in the cancer ward waiting for death.

JUST ONE VICTIM

I recently had the misfortune to witness something that will live in my mind forever. As most readers know, I spend my time doing radio and T.V. shows and visiting cancer clinics.

I was at one such clinic the other day. A young man of nineteen had thought it "cool" to smoke; he thought it made him look tough — and because he smoked a lot and took such big drags, he was accepted by his peers as a real cool character.

Not so when I saw him, however.

He had contacted cancer of the tongue.

The cobalt treatments had made things worse for him, and his tongue was so tender that it hurt to talk. He had been prepped for the operation to remove his tongue entirely, but the drug had not taken yet. I heard his screams first, and when I looked around he was being wheeled down the corridor to the operating room. He was screaming, "Don't take me in there. Please don't take me in there." You see, he knew that once in that room, his tongue would be removed and, if he lived, he would never be able to do any more than drool and make strange noises. So much for being cool.

Another injection quieted him down. I did not wait any longer, but left the hospital.

Mentioned recently in a New York paper: "More than eighty thousand deaths each year are caused by infections caught while in the hospital."

According to the "American College of Obstetricians and Gynecologists, "Up to 90,000 Caesarean sections could be avoided each year, considerably reducing the risk of maternal death, as well as length and cost of hospitalization." (Dr. Robert Cefalo, Committee Chairman, U.S. News and World Report, March 22, 1982.)

Not too long ago, a medical doctor in New York stated on television that, "over one hundred and fifty thousand unnecessary operations are performed each year in America.

Are Americans deprived of natural remedies commonly accepted and used in other countries? They most certainly are. Fortunately, the organization known as the "National Health Federation," Monrovia, California is fighting tooth and nail to remedy this.

Their fight on behalf of Laetrile, Perisel®, Enzymes, DMSO, Chelation, Jason Winter's Tribalene capsules and Freedom of Choice is well known.

Americans are told, for instance, that D.M.S.O. is worthless, and yet ...

In the year 1808 Russian lumberjacks, working in below freezing weather, discovered that if they rubbed D.M.S.O. (a product of trees) on their aching joints, the pain would quickly leave. Swollen arthritis would also disappear.

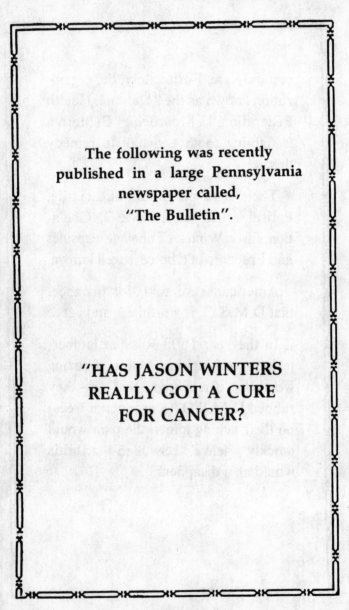

The following was recently
published in a large Pennsylvania
newspaper called,
"The Bulletin".

"HAS JASON WINTERS
REALLY GOT A CURE
FOR CANCER?

"In the past few years a lot of attention has been given to one man's extraordinary solution to the terrible dilemma of cancer. His name is Jason Winters and the special capsules which he formulated has been sold worldwide to millions of enthusiastic believers.

"This formula is now marketed in the form of capsules for greater convenience. Unlike the ordinary herb tablets manufactured by other competitors, Perisel Intl. who produces the unique Winters' formula have somehow been able to turn out a product that can be easily crushed between the thumb and forefinger with very little effort to say the least. Try and do that with a regular herb tablet. In most cases, considerable pressure has to be used to even make the darn thing disintegrate properly in your hand. And in a few other instances, a hammer must be employed to pulverize the tablet to powder.

"But not so with the Winters' capsule. If it can be rubbed with minimal ease into powder by the fingertips, just think how much more easily it can be assimilated into the digestive system. It would not be far-fetched at all to say that the capsule actually begins its immediate disintegration the moment it is swallowed and starts travelling down the alimentary canal to the stomach. No other herb tablet can work this swiftly.

"The all important question to ask however, is, "Does Tribalene really cure cancer?" By examining its simple ingredients, we can learn the answer to this ourselves.

"Its first and most significant ingredient is, of course, chaparral. Well over a decade, this remarkable shrub captured the attention of the medical world for its extraordinary ability to cause some tumor regression in some (but not all) forms of cancer. The literature proving this is too abundant to cite for lack of ample space here, but suffice it to say, this herb has been more closely looked at for its strong anti-cancer properties than many plants of late have been. A man who has used this herb, wrote to me sometime ago of how it benefitted him. Mr. Andrew Hanson of Oakland, Calif., testified that chaparral had successfully 'arrested' his leukemia. Another lady from Tempe, Arizona, Mrs. Kathalyn Windes, has also contacted me several times about the great value which this shrub has in the management of cancer. In neither case did the parties just mentioned, use the word 'cure'; but they did speak about the 'arrest' and proper 'management' of various kinds of malignant cancers in a responsible and truthful way.

"One could easily make claims for the Jason Winters' formula in the cure of cancer. I'm quite sure that there are those who would be willing to testify under oath that Tribalene has indeed cured them of one of Nature's most ravaging diseases.

But, if you're like me, then you prefer that which is closer to reality. That's why I feel comfortable with the words 'arrest' and 'properly manage' when describing the effects which Jason Winters' Tribalene can have on various kinds of cancer. After all, if it worked for Jason, then why shouldn't it work for someone else, too?

"Jason's other common ingredient is red clover. Jethro Kloss, America's greatest herbalist of the twentieth century, continually stressed the use of this fine herb throughout his book and especially in those sections where cancer is specifically mentioned. Of this wonderful herb, Jethro wrote: 'Red Clover is one of God's greatest blessings to man. I have used red clover blossoms for many years with excellent results. When I was a boy, my parents had me gather it for their postmaster who had a serious cancer. He lived to be an old man, without an operation.' (*Back To Eden, p.301*).

"The final ingredient that makes up the unique Winters' package is a rare herb from Southeast Asia, which Jason has romantically dubbed 'herbaline'. This precious spice not only gives the tea a different flavor but actually enhances the performances of the other 2 herbs and makes them work better. This synergistic effect is only achieved in the Winters' formula. Other competitors have sought to imitate his formula with blends of their own, but to no real avail. Perisel Intl., who Jason has officially authorized to manufacture his formula spend the majority of their time with just his products alone. Unlike their other competitors, they can devote a lot of attention to turning out a high-quality product. But when other companies that already carry dozens and dozens of single herbs and combinations get into the act, it's mostly for monetary reasons. Why should they spend a lot of unnecessary manufacturing time to something so special as this, when they've got an entire line of products to worry about. So they just crank out a cheap imitation of the real thing and peddle it along with the rest of their wares.

"Unfortunately, such unethical practices as this are to be expected in the free enterprise system. This is why Jason and the people who make his products, have affixed his portrait, signature and Perisel Intl. to the Winters' formula they make. This is to assure buyers of the genuine article and not some phoney reproductions.

"When you consider what Tribalene contains, it is no wonder that so many people speak well of it in the health field today. Chaparral has been proven scientifically. And besides that, famous Amish writers such as William McGrath have spoken highly of the herb, too. In his 'Mountaineer Commentary' column of June 27, 1979, in *The Budget,* McGrath not only praises chaparral for cancer but also specifically makes reference to Jason himself.

"Thus, while we may refrain from using the definitive word 'cure' to describe Jason Winter Tribalene, yet we can say, with all honesty and sincerity that it *does* 'arrest' and 'manage' various kinds of cancer, not to mention all of the other wonderful health benefits it can also yield."

The following is taken from the writings of Mr. Carl Richards, England's oldest living person, 113 years of age:

"Looking into Mr. Winters' report on Perisel® brought back memories of the time I resided in Lhasa, Tibet. I lived there from 1930 to 1938 and learned many of their health habits. Since that time I have consumed daily both the substances that Jason Winters has joined together, Gotu Kola, Spice and Selenium.

"I found that they must be taken in exact proportions, which always proved a difficulty, but now, with the advent of Perisel®, they are both measured correctly and placed in tablet form. I thank Jason Winters for doing something so wonderful, yet so simple. It has been said that the greatest breakthroughs will be the simplest ones, and Perisel® is no exception. I believe that these ingredients are necessary to maintain life, and today so many people are drastically lacking them that they are leading what I call 'half lives'. I am alive today because I visited the Himalayas and Tibet and learned these truths. Now Jason Winters is doing what I should have done forty-five years ago, and that is to make this knowledge available to everyone."

Carl Richards
London

HOPE IS
YOUR MOST VALUABLE ASSET

The medical profession's biggest argument against any alternative therapy, including laetrile, enzymes, D.M.S.O., Jason Winters Tribalene, any herbs, nutrition, faith, etc. is that it gives a patient false hope.

There is no such thing as False Hope. One of the wisdoms learned in Tibet is that words spoken to a sick person are like a weapon. Words spoken by a person's God-like doctor are taken for granted to be true.

How many times have you heard a doctor say,"We've done all we can, the rest is up to the patient. He must have the will to live."

The doctor is saying, in effect, that if the person has the will to live, then their chances are much better. Why is it then, especially in the case of cancer, that doctors send people home with "just three months to live"?

Don't they realize that just by saying that, they actually cause it to happen? They have taken away all hope, have superceded even Jesus when he said, "Faith can move mountains."

Tibetans believe that if a person has faith and hope, his body manufactures certain chemicals that aid in the curing. But if the patient is convinced that he will die, then his body manufactures chemicals to fulfill his belief.

Every religion in the world says it. Even our parents and school teachers said it: *If you want to do something bad enough, nothing can stop you.*

History books are full of people who won out against all odds. Every hero that we have ever heard of did this, and every man, woman, and child is capable of "winning out" regardless of their circumstances.

This is what the famous book *"The Power of Positive Thinking"* was all about. It's what the Bible is all about.

If you have an inferiority complex, you go to a psychiatrist and he tells you over and over again (under hypnosis) that you are as good, if not better than anyone else. Finally you believe it, and so you are cured.

If you constantly tell a child he is stupid, then eventually he believes it and so acts stupid. Encourage the same child every day by saying he is bright and will achieve, and he will. It is all so simple, yet the medical profession still keeps on handing out death sentences.

I believe that when a person is very ill, they hang on to every word their doctor utters. I have seen the excitement that rushes through a person's body when the doctor says, "You're going to be all right."

I have seen the person fall apart and die quickly when the doctor pronounces the death sentence. All of us must be careful of the words spoken to the sick. Jesus says that miracles can happen. So how can we dare, even if we are the most educated and intelligent doctor in the land, to call Jesus a liar and to thereby quicken the death by weeks, months, or maybe years?

The Miracle of Pure Water

The sun shines on the sea and lakes, causing vapour to rise and form clouds. This vapour is pure. It leaves behind all bacteria and, what's even more important, inorganic minerals. Inorganic minerals can not be used by the body. Rain water, traveling over lime stone and other minerals in the ground carry these minerals to plant life. The plants, vegetables, fruits, etc., then use these inorganic minerals for food, changing them into organic minerals. This is when the human body can use them to advantage. These are the minerals necessary for our good health.

Rain water is no longer pure because it has to fall through layers of filthy air, and because distilled water acts as a magnet for toxic materials, by the time it hits land it is also toxic.

Hard water, or any water other than distilled water, is full of lime salts, calcium, magnesium, sodium, iron, copper, silicon, nitrates, chlorides, viruses, bacteria, chemicals, and many other inorganic materials detrimental to the body. Over five billion tons of dissolved minerals are washed into the sea every year. Because of this, sea life has been reduced fifty percent over the last thirty years. Pesticides and factory waste are responsible for most of this.

Many thousands of people are under the false impression that bottled water or filtered water keeps them safe. Treated bottled water does kill the bacteria, but does not remove the minerals that are just as harmful.

If you have a private filter that you use, it still only removes bacteria, leaving the harmful minerals. Plus, some experts say that a filter only works well for the first two days, then turns into a breeding ground for bacteria, thereby defeating its own purpose. Also, experts say, treated bottled water is full of dead bacteria, which, although not directly causing illness, does definitely set the groundwork, entering the body and eventually acts as a compost heap or fertilizer for bacteria to grow and spread.

The idea of drinking water was originally to flush poisons from the body, washing every cell daily. Each living cell in our body is a life of its own. It needs to take nourishment from the blood and to expell poisons. Imagine, if you will, that inorganic minerals that you have been consuming since birth in your water supply have surrounded almost every cell of your body, making it impossible for the cell to do its job properly, if at all. This is degeneration, illness and death, not only to that particular cell, but to you as a person

Throw drinking water on a glass or mirror, and when it dries you are left with spots. That is the inorganic minerals that are even now surrounding each cell, making it difficult to live a normal healthy life. Take distilled water and do the same. You will find that it leaves no spots at all.

Well water is every bit as harmful, but there is good news at last. Start drinking distilled water, and only distilled water. It makes everything taste better. Also, it acts as a magnet in your body, leeching out all of those harmful minerals that have been accumulating around every cell since the day you were born. It washes every cell and, I think, because of the thousands of testimonies I have read, will do away with aging and most ills. Water distillers are available in many sizes, and we consider ours as the most important appliance in our home, making our lives so vibrant and happy. Try distilled water for one month and you won't believe the results. Perisel works well, but with distilled water it is dynamite. Every group in the world, known for longevity, has access to pure water with no minerals. It truly is a Godsend.

The water distiller that I purchased, after much investigation, was from Durastill P.O.Box 76641-W Atlanta, Georgia 30328. They are a wonderful company that will send you all information upon request.

15 THE LOWDER COLONIC BOARD

I had just finished reading the famous book "BACK TO EDEN" written by that most brilliant herbalist, Jethro Kloss. I had been particularly interested in page 144, explaining high enemas. It was made abundantly clear to me that whatever a person does to regain their health, it doesn't mean a thing if you have a dirty colon.

I had lunch that day with Eldon Lowder, and mentioned to him about the importance of the colon. He perked up immediately and for the rest of the meal spoke at great lengths about rotting fecal matter lodged in peoples colons sometimes for 20 years. He said the colon was the cause of most disease, being dark, damp and warm, a perfect breeding ground. He wondered why I didn't order desert, then said, "I have designed a perfect high colonic board which people are raving over. It is strong and comfortable and allows people to thoroughly clean their colon with ease, in the privacy of their own bathroom." I was surprised because I had always thought that this cleansing had to be done by a professional.

He told me of a friend whom had thought he was healthy but decided to try Eldon's colonic board. On the third time of using, the friend called Eldon to say that he had passed particularly viscious looking worms. Eldon then reached across the table to ask if I would like to finish up with some hot chocolate, which I refused. He continued that because of the curved design of the board, there was no splashback, therefore eliminating the threat of vaginal infections. I now own one of these specially designed colonic boards, and in all honesty I must admit that, in spite of all the enemas I had taken since terminal cancer, I was very surprised at the results. To know that you have a clean colon is very reassuring. Eldon Lowder is most successful today, and ships his colonic boards far and wide. I recommend that everyone contact him and obtain a board of their own. It just stands in a closet while not in use.

To avoid a thousand letters, I will give his address here.

Eldon Lowder
Western Health Research
7835 S. 1300 E.
Sandy, Utah 84092

(If you happen to read this, Mr. Lowder, I must say that I may not have enjoyed the lunch, but I am sincerely thankful for the information you gave me, that has since helped so many, God bless you.)

WARNING: Please do not buy any Jason Winters Products from any source (including health food stores) until you contact Jason Winters. Crooks are already cashing in on your misfortune by selling useless products & using Jason Winters name & photo.

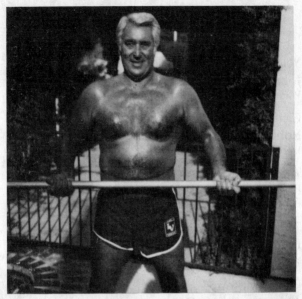

Jason Winters today, five years after he should have died. He lifts weights each day and is entering over forty weightlifting tournaments in 1983.

Everything Winters drinks is made with distilled water. Jason says "For the finest water distiller available today," contact the good people at DURASTILL, INC., P.O. Box 76641 "W", Atlanta, GA 30328.

Great Books to Read

Your Body Doesn't Lie"
John Diamond, M.D.
Warner Books

Confessions of a Medical Heretic
Robert S. Mendelsohn M.D.
Warner Books

Threshold To Tomorrow
Ruth Montgomery
Putnam Publishers

The Essene Gospel of Peace
Edmond Bordeaux Szekely

New Age Companion
Peggy Mason
43A Broadwater Down
Tunbridge Wells
Kent
England.

Back to Eden
Jethro Kloss
Jethro Kloss Family
P.O. Box 1439
Loma Linda, CA 92354

The Vitamin Bible
Earl Mindell

The Subtle Body
David V. Tansley

Should wish to contact Jason Winters directly, please write to:

> Jason Winters
> 4055 S. Spencer St.
> Suite 227
> Las Vegas, Nevada 89109

If you are like so many other readers of this remarkable book, you will want to order one for a friend. Please try your local health food store for a copy, as many of the better stores carry it.

If you cannot obtain a copy locally, then please fill out the order form below.

SEND CHEQUE or MONEY ORDER

Please rush me:
☐ KILLING CANCER at $5.95 each

Name _____

Address_____

City_____ State_____ Zip_____

Signature _____

Add sales tax where applicable

VINTON PUBLISHING
1244 Wyoming Street
Boulder City, Nevada 89005

The old man squatted in the dust beside me, and as we gazed down the street of cages in Bombay, he began to speak. "You see, my son, this life is an illusion—It simply prepares us for the real life in spirit — The eternal, everlasting, ever concious life beyond the grave. Without loss of awareness we are there, free, happy and painless, happy in the complete knowledge that life is everlasting."

His sparkling eyes shone from amidst a thousand wrinkles, and he whispered "This great truth is hidden from man for fear he may try to reach the spirit world too soon. He must do his schooling on earth first."

Tears came to my eyes as I realized that I had always known this truth. Deep inside, we all do.